ADVANCED
THETAHEALING®

ADVANCED THETAHEALING®

Harnessing the Power of
All That Is

Vianna Stibal

HAY HOUSE, INC.
Carlsbad, California • New York City
London • Sydney • Johannesburg
Vancouver • Hong Kong • New Delhi

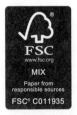
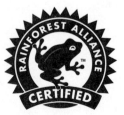

Contents

From the Editor: To our readers in the U.S. and Canada, please note that for the most part, we have maintained the British style of spelling, grammar (including noun/pronoun agreement), punctuation, and syntax of the most recent printing of this book, which was published in the United Kingdom.

FOREWORD

I am living testimony to the purity of this work. This information came from conversations with the Creator and thousands of readings and healings, not to mention interaction with Vianna's students and instructors and ThetaHealing® classes over a period of years. The ideas and processes were spontaneous in their formulation and never devised through the abuse of information from other established or unestablished energy-healing modalities. The definitive sources and resources that are used in ThetaHealing are available to all who wish to know.

Springing from a conservative community in America, ThetaHealing has become a world-wide healing modality. In view of the considerable challenges that were experienced in its formulation, I am constantly amazed at how it has triumphed. Against all probability, it has indeed become a light in the darkness, a gift from the divine.

There have been many people, all in their own way, who have contributed to making ThetaHealing the energy-healing modality that it has become. These are the clients, students, practitioners and certified instructors who, in varying degrees, have made contributions that cannot be overlooked. Nevertheless, no matter how many people have been involved in ThetaHealing, no matter how many people have taken these teachings into themselves, the inescapable fact still remains that it all came from the resolve, bravery and pure faith of one person: *Vianna*.

Having witnessed the development first-hand, I can comfortably say that I have never seen such truth, faith and determination in a human being as I have in Vianna. To me, this is why she is the loving leader of ThetaHealing and the only person qualified to be so. I believe that this is why the information comes through her. Many people love God, but I have seen few stand in the light and presence of the divine with such conviction that God the Creator is *real*.

The contents of this book come from Vianna's visionary and physical experiences. It is offered as a guide to the ability of the mind to heal through the Creator of All That Is. The rest is up to you and your beliefs.

Guy Stibal

PREFACE

Advanced ThetaHealing is the companion to the books *ThetaHealing* and *ThetaHealing: Diseases and Disorders*. In the first book, *ThetaHealing*, I explain the step-by-step processes of the ThetaHealing reading, healing, belief work, feeling work, digging and gene work, and offer an introduction to the planes of existence and additional knowledge for the beginner. This book provides an in-depth guide to belief, feeling and digging work and further insights into the planes of existence and the beliefs that I believe are essential for spiritual evolution. It does not include all the specific step-by-step processes that proliferate in *ThetaHealing*, though it is necessary to reach an understanding of these processes in order to fully utilize this book.

ThetaHealing is a process of meditation that creates physical, psychological and spiritual healing using the *Theta* brainwave. While in a pure and divine Theta state of mind, we are able to connect with the Creator of All That Is thorough focused prayer.

There is one requirement that is absolute with this technique: you must have a central belief in the Creator. The name is of lesser importance – I realize that the Creator has many different names, and God, Buddha, Shiva, Goddess, Jesus, Yahweh and Allah are all currents leading in a flow towards the Seventh Plane of Existence and the Creative Energy of All That Is. ThetaHealing has no religious affiliation. Neither are its processes specific to any age, sex, race, colour, creed or religion. Anyone with a pure belief in God or the creative force can access and use the branches of the ThetaHealing tree.

The Creator has given us the fascinating knowledge you are about to receive. It is a compilation of information from the DNA advanced classes, the *DNA 2 Advanced Manual* and recordings, and is the prelude to DNA 3.

Even though I am sharing this information with you, I do not accept any responsibility for the changes that can arise from its use. That responsibility is yours, a responsibility you assume when you realize that you have the power to change your life as well as the lives of others.

Acknowledgements

I would like to thank all the wonderful clients and students who gave me the opportunity to learn the information that has finally come to rest here. This manuscript focuses on the experiences of belief work encountered in some of the thousands of sessions I have done. May this knowledge be a gift to all those brave souls out there who dare to *believe*.

INTRODUCTION

Hello, I am Vianna.

On a dark moonless night in 2003, I was driving down the long road from work towards my home in the country. Suddenly I had a most amazing epiphany. I realized that it had been nine years since the beginning of my journey in ThetaHealing and I had come a long way. During those nine years, I had given thousands of readings and healings, taught numerous classes and written books on the ThetaHealing technique. But I had learned one undeniable truth: I still had much to learn.

Driving down that lonely road along the Snake river, I heard the voice of the Creator telling me that I had finished my nine-year indentured service and would be entering a three-year period of being a teacher. I would be teaching the preparation for DNA 3, ThetaHealing for advanced students. This alarmed me a little, because every time new ThetaHealing information had begun to come to me, there had been great changes in my life. However, I calmed myself down and said, 'OK, God, what is DNA 3 all about?'

I was told that DNA 3 would involve the knowledge of how to move and change organic and non-organic matter, as well as how to work with mitochondria to create instant healing. I had already experienced instant manifestations and healings, as had others close to me, so this didn't surprise me.

I was told that when 100 people understood the advanced information, implementing its concepts would be much easier, as the ability to do so would spread through the collective consciousness of humanity. I would know when 100 people truly understood it, and when 1,000 people believed in, knew and lived it, the advanced knowledge itself would spread throughout our collective consciousness and escalate the awakening of our latent abilities.

I was told, 'First you believe in the concepts, then you know them and then you live within them. The advanced information will open neural pathways that have never been awake before.'

When I heard this, I couldn't help but wish that the mundane challenges of my everyday life could be more like my work. Doing readings and healings and being inside the human body were where I was most comfortable, moving around cells and bone in the blissful state of Theta. It was when I was *outside* the body dealing with everyday stress that things became strange.

In answer to this wish, the Creator explained:

'Vianna, in or out of Theta, in or out of the body, it is all the same. How many people think about the body's functions as they run its internal systems? At any one time there are numerous electrical impulses from the brain to the body that tell it to breathe, to grow, to feel hunger, to digest food and all the other unconscious acts that go on. In much the same way, the brain and the soul are connected to the giant nervous system of the Earth. The Earth in turn is connected to the nervous system of the universe, our infinite "outside" body. This outer connection to the universe is the same as our inner connection to the body in that we may effect changes upon the universe outside our space in much the same way as we do internally. The reason this is not happening today is because centuries of children were raised with the beliefs that they had limitations. And we have accepted these limitations in, around and through the DNA on the spiritual, mental, emotional and physical levels.'

It was at that moment that I began to have a deeper understanding of the Creator's plan for the ThetaHealing information and how it was to be relayed and implemented.

You see, when I was given the belief and feeling work, I was shown that we all had the capability to dissolve our limitations and be truly connected to the God-Self that is within all of us. I understood that as a species it had taken us centuries to collect these limitations, or 'programmes', on physical, emotional, mental and spiritual levels. Without a means of releasing them, it would take centuries to get rid of them. In the past, this was how we evolved – level by level, generation by generation and life by life. We only evolved a little during each lifetime so that we could understand everything that particular life had to give. But now, through *spiritual evolution*, I realized we were developing the ability to look beyond the confines of our reality and open ourselves to other aspects of creation. We were being given a way to eliminate *in this life* the belief systems that no longer served us.

I now know we all have the opportunity to reach a new stage of development where we will be given the keys to unlock the floodgates to the dam that has prevented our 'karma' from moving forward. Genetics, disease, childhood programmes, energetic influences and issues from the collective consciousness have all kept us from developing to our full potential as co-creators with the Creator of All That Is. But now we can avoid being affected by the choices of our ancestors and even the influences of our present-day lives. It is time to begin to use our power as divine sparks of God.

In this book I present to you the preparation for DNA 3, advanced ThetaHealing, that has been taught since 2003. The golden rule of advanced ThetaHealing is to be careful with this work. Once your intuitive abilities have developed, it is imperative that you are conscious of the thought forms you project while in a Theta state. This is why it is important to use the belief work to remove and replace negative programmes in addition to downloading feelings from the Creator to bring yourself to a place of purity in your thoughts.

Your mind is incredible. It moves your body with electrical impulses. With these techniques you will learn to use the electrical impulses that move things *outside* the body, too. You must also develop the wisdom to use your abilities without fear and to know the difference between your emotions and the *truth*.

Most of the students and instructors who are doing Theta work are wonderful people. However, occasionally there may be an individual who is unbalanced or overly egotistical; that is simply the way life can be. This is one of the reasons for presenting the advanced information. This information is designed to sort the people who should be doing Theta work from those who should not.

Always remember, *free will* is a wonderful gift, but it should not interfere with the *free agency* of another person.

In 2002 I had a dream that I now see pertained to this subject. In the dream I had been given the job of protecting a baby. There was a mystery surrounding this child. At first I thought that someone was trying to kill it, since everyone who came close to it was cut to shreds. I would walk into the room just as something terrible was happening to someone and I realized that it was the baby that was the cause. You see, it had too much uncontrolled psychic power, so anyone who made it angry or upset was cut into ribbons. That baby was a symbol of our psychic abilities run wild, of our misuse and ignorance of our abilities, much like the person who drives down the street sending curses out to anyone in their way. The child was incredibly intuitive, but had not gained wisdom along with power. It had not had time to develop wisdom.

The moral of this story is that if you have power without wisdom, it is possible to misuse it. In this space and time many people have belief programmes that *will* cause them to misuse the abilities that come with ThetaHealing. These programmes may be held on different belief levels. For some people, self-sabotaging programmes exist on an unconscious level. In other instances, a practitioner's negative ego may be limiting their development as a ThetaHealer®. Balance is the key to becoming an intuitive healer using energy work. If the healer is unbalanced, it is possible that the readings and healings will not be effective.

Unconditional love must also be projected in readings, healings and the teaching of this work. If you do not truly *love* the people you are healing, they can sense it. If you look inward and find that you dislike certain people, perhaps you should use the belief work until you see the *truth* about people and still accept and *love* them for who they are. We might recognize traits in others that we find annoying, but it is the mastership of those traits within *ourselves* that will overcome the endless circle of competition in the world. Releasing bottom beliefs and accepting essential feelings from the Creator will set you free.

Welcome to Advanced ThetaHealing!

The very nature of life can be perceived as pure energy. The seven planes of existence are the dance and the circle of this energy. This divine energy is never-ending, simply changing form through different frequencies of vibration. No plane of existence is more important than any other. The objective is to become balanced with the energy of every plane through the Seventh Plane of the Creator of All That Is, the universal spirit that animates and binds all things in existence.

The purpose of this book is not only to explain this but to focus on the energy that brings the best and quickest results and to show that what is created can be 'dis-created' and then re-created again.

Advanced ThetaHealing is the understanding of the spiritual nature of atoms and the knowledge that we are magnificent beings creating reality.

1

REVIEWING THETAHEALING FEELING WORK

In this book you will to learn how to heal from the *Seventh Plane of Existence*. This is the *essence of All That Is*.

You will also learn more details about all of the planes, how to eliminate oaths, vows and commitments that are no longer serving you and how to heal broken souls.

You will bring in feelings that you may never have experienced before.

You will clear space in the mind that is wasted holding on to random negative emotions such as anger, revenge, resentment, regret, aggression, jealousy, envy and bitterness. This will allow you to utilize more energy, to achieve faster healings, to advance the human species and to connect to the divine.

Before beginning this book, please understand that you are responsible for your own decisions and your own life. The concepts laid out here are wonderful and will help you grow, but cannot be used to override another person's free will. No matter who you are, no matter what you think, the truth is that we are *all* here to learn by experience and that we *all* have free will. Free will is a Law of the Universe. It just is. If you are reading this book with other ideas in mind, then perhaps this information isn't for you. Anyone who uses this work and abuses it must understand that there are other Laws that are connected to free will, such as the Law of Truth and the Law of Justice. To break a Law such as free will would mean being in direct opposition to the Law of Truth and the Law of Justice. All the Laws work synergistically with one another to enhance the attributes that are inherent in each individual Law. This is something that is essential to bear in mind as you carry out this work.

❖❖❖❖❖

In 2003 I was told that there would be a DNA 3 ThetaHealing class. In order to advance to this class and understand and utilize the information, students would need certain downloads (feelings they might never have

1

known) from the Creator of All That Is. These downloads were offered in what came to be called the Advanced ThetaHealing class and are in this book. This book teaches you how to download these feelings into yourself by accessing the highest definition of them from the Creator of All That Is. I understand that many of you will already have some of these feelings and beliefs and may not experience Earth-shattering changes as a result of downloading them. However, understanding these feelings properly can create positive changes in your life.

This is how we believe it works: from the point of conception up to the present time, our cells have been trained in what to expect in the way of messages coming in through their receptors. Every cell has receptors. They are there to receive nutrition, hormones and communication. They act as receiving, docking and distribution points so the cells can function.

The cells have also been trained, from the time that we were very young, by the *emotional* messages that have been sent to them. If you grew up in a household in which most of the family was chronically depressed, for example, you may have receptors that are designed to cause you to be chronically depressed. As you grow older, this will eventually create a situation where the cells of the body will not feel normal unless you are depressed. In fact, you may not feel normal unless you become depressed about something at least once a day. In this situation, the body has been trained to be chronically depressed through the influence of family members.

In order to assist a person with depression using ThetaHealing, we might use belief work, as explained in my first book. However, pulling the belief of 'I am depressed' and replacing it with another programme may not clear the issue. This is where the feeling work comes in. What must be done in this instance is to teach the body in the highest and best way *how to live without depression*. This retrains the receptors to shut the tiny doorways that permit the messages for depression to enter in and to open new pathways into the cell for beneficial emotions and feelings. When you insert a new feeling programme, these new receptor pathways will be created at the same time. So now the cell understands how to live without depression. And changes in the cells are recorded in the DNA, so when the cell replicates itself, the new cell will also have the new pathways.

As well as changing the receptors on the cells with feeling work, when we introduce a new concept or modify a certain belief, new neuronal circuits are created in the brain. The brain is a biological electromagnetic transmitter and receiver of information – a characteristic that allows us to learn. For example, if you release the programme of believing you are ugly and replace it with believing you are beautiful, the neurons will follow a new pattern. However, you must first know what it *feels like* to be beautiful.

2

In most instances, the *digging technique* must precede the insertions of feelings or the release of programmes. This technique enables us to understand which neuronal connections we need to change. Then we have to make sure that we change any associated patterns that might interfere with the new concept. In my first book I discuss digging for the bottom beliefs. In this book, I will give a more in-depth explanation of the process.

Digging does not mean asking the Creator what to change and nothing more. It involves a discussion with the client, since the simple act of talking about the topic will free them from part of their issue. It will, in effect, bring the programmes into the light of the conscious mind to be released spontaneously. The key point is in the client–practitioner interaction, but the client must not focus too much on the idea that their brain is being reprogrammed or the subconscious may attempt to replace the new programme with the old one.

When you encounter a new programme connected to a receptor, ask the Creator whether to release it, replace it or simply delete some aspect of it. Never replace programmes without proper discernment. What may at first be perceived as a negative programme may actually be beneficial. Programmes should not be randomly released.

Teaching the subconscious to behave differently is not a novel idea of my own. Many people use different processes, such as reading the same thing for 30 days, to change the subconscious mind. In ThetaHealing, however, we believe the changes are almost instantaneous. Beliefs are pulled, sent to the Creator, replaced with new programmes and feelings instilled from the Creator, and there you are. We believe that by using the belief and feeling work it is possible to make physical changes to the body and heal disease. I have watched many lives change simply through downloading feelings from the Creator.

2

DISCOVER THE SEVENTH PLANE

As I teach people in ThetaHealing classes, I observe them not only in the physical sense, but in the numinous sense as well. I use an intuitive visual awareness that permits me to see where they are going with their consciousness when they do the exercises. Remember, in ThetaHealing we imagine going up out of our space to trigger a Theta brainwave, which is why ThetaHealing works. But it didn't take me long to realize that everyone seemed to be going to different places.

During one of these classes, one of my students, frustrated with her results, asked me where *I* was going to co-create readings and healings. I told her the best way that I could, but I realized that the process had become so natural to me that words couldn't easily do it justice. Yet somehow I had to put it into words. This motivated me to sit down and write down the process step by step in what became known as *the road map to the Seventh Plane*.

I have outlined this process already in *ThetaHealing*, but I will go through it again here as it is only by going up to the Seventh Plane that you can tap into the creative energy of All That Is. It is here that the energy of creation exists, so you can 'dis-create' illness and re-create health in an instant. It is where ThetaHealers should be going to and healing from.

When you imagine yourself going up out of your space to the Seventh Plane, you are leaving behind your personal paradigm and limited perceptions of the world. This process will trigger new pathways to all parts of the brain and almost turn your consciousness inside out, enabling you to look at everything around you with clarity.

GOING UP TO THE SEVENTH PLANE

The following process is given to you by the Creator to train All That You Are to connect to and understand All That Is. Once this is learned, you will consistently go to the Seventh Plane and will not need to go through the whole process, as you will simply recognize that you are already there.

4

Imagine energy coming up through the bottom of your feet from the centre of the Earth and going up out of the top of your head as a beautiful ball of light. You are in this ball of light. Take time to notice what colour it is.

Now imagine going up above the universe.

Now imagine going into the light above the universe. It is a big beautiful light.

Imagine going up through that light, and you will see another bright light, and another, and another. In fact there are many bright lights. Keep going. Between the lights there is a little bit of dark light, but this is just a layer before the next light, so keep going.

Finally there is a great big bright gold light. Go through it. Then you will see a jelly-like substance that has all the colours of the rainbow in it. When you go into it, you will see that it changes colour. This is the Laws. You will see all kinds of shapes and colours here.

In the distance, there is a white iridescent light. It is a white-blue colour, like a pearl. Head for that light. Avoid the deep blue light you will see, because this is the Law of Magnetism.

As you get closer to the iridescent light, you will see a pink mist. Keep going until you see it. This is the Law of Compassion, and it will push you towards the light.

You will see that the iridescent light is in the shape of a rectangle, like a window. This window is really the opening to the Seventh Plane. Go through it and deep within it. See a deep, whitish glow go through your body. Feel it. It feels light, but it has essence. You can feel it going through you and it's as if you can no longer feel any separation between your own body and the energy. You become All That Is. Don't worry. Your body will not disappear. It may become perfect and healthy. Remember there is just energy here, not people or things. So if you see people, go higher.

It is from this place that the Creator of All That Is can perform instant healing and that you can create in all aspects of your life.

Practise using this way of going to the Seventh Plane of Existence. It will unlock doors ins your mind and stimulate neurons in your brain to connect you to the energy of creation. It doesn't take you out to the far-flung universe; rather, it takes you to an inner part of your being that you may have not experienced before, your inner universe. This is why some people see a mirror image of themselves when they first go to the Seventh Plane.

Where you are truly going is to the beginning of all things. And there you will realize that you are connected to *everything*.

THE EXPANDING METHOD

Another way of reaching the Seventh Plane is through the expanding method. This should not be tried until you have had experience with the first method and have therefore realized that there is energy all around you and you are an integral part of All That Is.

Seat yourself in a comfortable chair or sofa and take a deep breath in. Imagine that you and the chair have become one on a molecular level. Your molecules and those of the chair are transferring back and forth. You are connecting to the molecules, becoming as one with them.

Now imagine that on a molecular level you are a part of everything in the room. Expand outward and become as one with the outside world.

Imagine that you are a part of the area, then the country that you are in.

Imagine that you are a part of the entire Earth, connecting to Earth, land and sea, every creature, every nation on this planet, until you and the Earth are one and the same.

Imagine that you and the universe are one and the same.

Imagine that you are a part of all the bright white lights.

Imagine that you are a part of the jelly-like substance.

Finally imagine that you are a part of an iridescent white light that is the Seventh Plane of Existence. Become as one with this iridescent white light, it tingles.

Take a deep breath in and open your eyes. Welcome to the Seventh Plane of Existence. For behold, you are not separate, you are a part of God – All That Is.

TAKING A SHORTCUT

Once you have gone through this process, you will find you will be able to go to the Seventh Plane instantly by commanding that you are there. It is a switch that is tripped in the brain.

Remember, you are going to the Seventh *Plane*, not to the seventh *level*. There are many levels within the planes of existence and if you were to command to go to the seventh level you would be going to the Fifth Plane.

GROUNDING

When you come back from the Seventh Plane and bring your consciousness back into your space, there is a proper way to *ground back into yourself*. It is important that you once again send your energy-consciousness down into the centre of the Earth, then bring it back into your space.

When some people bring themselves back into their space after sending their consciousness into another person's space in a healing or reading, they do not filter their essence through the All That Is before they reconnect to their body. It is best to connect to the All That Is when you come back into your space.

THE CREATOR

Many people believe that what they are doing when they go to the Seventh Plane is ascending into the cosmos. What they are actually doing, as already explained, is triggering something *within themselves*, in the energy, the core and structure of an atom. This act is a soul remembrance that we are connected to the Creator of All That Is.

In many cultures, the Creator is thought to be male, or a male god. But when you reach the Seventh Plane you reach the energy that creates *All*. Here there is no male, no female, just the energy of creation that resides in us all.

One of my student teachers could never grasp the concept that the Creator was everywhere and that we were all a part of that Creator. I remember doing my best to take her up to the Seventh Plane so that she would understand. She burst into tears, telling me that it was too far, that the Creator was too far from her. I told her, 'Once you reach the Seventh Plane and open your eyes to the All That Is energy, you will see a reflection of yourself there.' But in all the time I was teaching that class, she never understood the concept. She never stopped wallowing in her old beliefs long enough to listen to what I was saying.

Part of the goal of ThetaHealing is to use the belief work to clear any blocks that keep you from realizing that you are reaching and *are part of* the Seventh Plane and the All That Is. This is the energy that you need to understand in order to use DNA 3.

CONNECTING TO THE DIVINE

It is also possible to go up and out with your consciousness to connect directly with the Creator. The best way I have found of doing it is as follows:

1. Begin beneath your feet and draw energy from the centre of the Earth.
2. Draw this energy up into yourself.

This automatically opens the chakras and activates the energy of *kundalini*. With this energy, the connection is made with the Creator of All That Is of the Seventh Plane of Existence.

It is important that this procedure is followed, because it opens the chakras and raises the *kundalini* safely and correctly. In my experience, if the *kundalini* is activated too quickly there is the possibility that it will strain the physical organs.

3

THE ADVANCED READING

Readings in ThetaHealing use the Theta brainwave, which has been found to have several interesting properties. Scientists have discovered that certain brain frequencies (particularly in the Alpha, Theta and Theta-Gamma ranges):

- alleviate stress and promote long-lasting and substantial reductions in anxiety

- facilitate deep physical relaxation and mental clarity

- increase verbal ability and verbal performance IQ

- synchronize both hemispheres of the brain

- invoke vivid spontaneous mental imagery and imaginative creative thinking, reduce pain, promote euphoria and stimulate endorphin release.

Every time you connect to the Creator of All That Is in a Theta state, you activate neurological pathways in the frontal lobe of your brain. This is the part that is activated when you get a placebo response. The more you maintain a Theta wave, the more developed that part of your brain becomes, leaving you feeling a little euphoric after you've been in Theta.

Maintaining the Theta wave may not be easy at first, but with practice an advanced practitioner of ThetaHealing will be able to maintain a Theta wave with 50 people in a room, on a crowded street or in the midst of any kind of noise or chaos. Obviously it is much easier to reach a divine meditative state in a peaceful and harmonic setting, but we do not always have this kind of luxury. What is important is to be able to use our intuitive abilities even in the midst of commotion. Our mind must be trained to shift to the divine Theta state instantly, before our conscious mind can talk us out of it with fears and doubts about our abilities.

THE READING

In order to train the brain to do a reading or healing, use the following process (this is a simplified version of a more elaborate and extensive process that the beginner is taught and that is given in *ThetaHealing*):

1. Begin in the heart chakra.
2. Send your energy down to the centre of Mother Earth.
3. Bring the energy back up into your body to open the chakras and create *kundalini*.
4. Send the energy up and out of your crown chakra.
5. Go through all the planes of existence using the road map to All That Is.
6. Make the connection to the Seventh Plane of Existence and the Creator of All That Is.
7. Make the command to witness the reading.
8. Go into the person's space and witness the inside of their body.
9. Once you have finished, move your consciousness out of their space through the crown chakra, disconnect by rinsing yourself off in a stream of water or white light and enter your body through your crown chakra. Send your consciousness down into Mother Earth to ground yourself and pull the energy up through your body to your crown.

Once this process becomes a thing of synchronistic spontaneity, you will not find it necessary to mechanistically go through a step-by-step process. In a timeless instant, the energy connection from the centre of the Earth will be sent up the spine to the crown chakra. With this Theta consciousness, you will go through all the planes of existence using the road map to the Creator. Then, in a timeless moment, you will unite with the divine energy of the Creator of All That Is of the Seventh Plane of Existence.

THE REWARD OF THE ROAD MAP

The road map serves as a focus for the consciousness and is intended in part to keep you from being distracted by the allure of the first six planes of existence. Also, within the process of the road map there is a hidden pattern of activation that will stimulate your brain and enhance your ability to perform readings and healings.

Continual use of the road map will help you to understand and use the energy of All That Is. This is, because each time you go up to the white lights, to the black lights and through the blackness to the brightest white light, different parts of your brain are 'switched on' to the seven planes and the Creator of All That Is.

As you feel yourself going up to the Creator, witness the activation of your frontal lobe, your pineal gland, your pituitary and your hypothalamus. A wave of energy will wash over these parts of the brain. As you use the road-map meditation, you will be exercising 'muscles' in the brain that you may not have used for a while.

You may ask, 'What is the reward for this?' It is that you'll find what you're looking for. You'll find a peace, a pureness and a joy that you cannot imagine. These feelings will stay with you. It will then be your responsibility to share them with some of the people around you (because it's nice to do that).

ASCENSION

I believe that when we ascend to the Seventh Plane, we are actually going on a journey inward *at the same time* as we are travelling outward into the infinities of Creation. We are journeying within our own brain to the message carriers, the neurons, and following the pathways of the neuronal circuits of the body to go within the very atomic energy that is in every molecule.

We are stimulated by an awareness – the awareness that we are connected to every molecule, every atom and the energy associated with subatomic particles. This is the first step in ascension. It will be this inner awareness that will bring us to the realization that we no longer have the need for the incredible competition that currently exists in the world, and the battle of duality will be over. The massive power of the universe is within us, waiting to coalesce within us. Once this power has been recognized within, through the focused Theta brainwave, it will flow outwards to the macrocosm of our everyday lives, expanding through the planes of existence to the immense macrocosm of the Creator of All That Is.

THE COMMAND

In ThetaHealing we are taught to make a *command* to our unconscious mind to do something. This is then witnessed through visualization. What we should realize is that in making this command we do not question, with either the conscious or unconscious mind, whether this will be done – this process removes all doubts about our own worthiness, abilities or otherwise. The command itself brings the realization of our own part in the healing.

However, we must not lose sight of what the command is and is not. We have to train ourselves to know the difference between a *command* and a *demand* when we communicate with the divine.

One of the most important things that ThetaHealing gives us is the ability to *communicate with* the divine – not *demand of* the divine. It is not designed to be used as a *wish list* for the smallest or most expansive of egotistical desires.

Also, ThetaHealing is not about talking *at* the Creator. It is about talking *to* the Creator and *listening* to the Creator. This is true communication with the divine.

WITNESSING THE COMMAND

It is through the *witnessing* of a healing or manifestation that the *command* will actually work. There is a Law that says *'If it is not witnessed, it won't happen.'*

I find that many healers get in a big hurry and leave the body before they finish witnessing the process. If you don't witness the process as complete, it won't *be* complete.

THE RINSING

The beginner is taught to rinse off any residual energy from the client with a stream of water or white light when they return to their own space. But when the advanced practitioner has reached a point of true communication it will not be necessary to rinse off the residual psychic energy. This is because the readings and healings will be done from the perfect energy of All That Is.

GENTLY, SOFTLY

A focused Theta brainwave that is filtered through the Creator is a very gentle signal and it is not necessary to 'act it out' with physical gestures. I have watched many of my students roll their eyes back in their head while doing readings or vibrate their whole body like a tuning fork. Some people even act as though they are having a difficult bowel movement! They are *all* trying too hard.

The best way to enter someone's space is to go in as gently as a feather floating on the breeze. Go in as though you were *a part* of their body, not *separate* from it. The body's systems have their own sentience, their own intelligence. The cells of the body can sense that your consciousness is in the body and if the macrophages perceive you as a threat, the immune system may start working harder than it should to counter a perceived attack from a foreign invader. So go in with the ultimate reverence – gently, softly and with permission. You are entering someone's holy temple.

FOCUS

When a person asks for a reading, you have to stay focused on their energy. However, if you are too busy being focused on being focused, you may miss something. Readings are all about focus *and* maintaining a Theta state.

Also, if you are going to do readings as a career, you need to know it's not always easy, because you are dealing with people and everyone is different. It does take discipline. When I began doing this work, I put it out to the universe that the Creator brought me people by word of mouth, but I always *showed up* for work. I went to work every day and waited for that phone to ring. I made sure that I played my part in the process.

I have heard people say, 'I don't want to do readings today. I'm not in the mood.' And then they wonder why they don't have a consistent clientèle. I made sure that I made myself available and showed up every day, even on nights and Saturdays if that was when the person had the time.

Some of my beginner students are terrified of being wrong in a reading. I can understand this. I have done thousands of readings, but right before I get on the phone or go into a session with a client, my heart still flutters a little with nervousness. Then I go up and connect to the Creator and everything is alright. I always know when I go into Theta that the Creator is going to take care of it.

I can't tell another person how long it will be before they have consistent and pure communication with the Creator. Everyone is going to be different, because we all have different belief systems.

One thing I do know is that after a long day of working with multiple clients, there will always be that one person that I am grateful to for giving me inspiration. I will say, 'Creator, thank you for bringing this person to me today.'

One of these people was a woman who was paralyzed due to multiple sclerosis. We worked on her belief systems, and by the time we had finished, it was as if she was the one who was giving me the therapy, not the other way around. She didn't say 'Can you heal me?' but 'What do I have to do to make the Creator proud of me?'

After an inspiring reading like this, everything comes back into perspective again and I'm high on these feelings for days.

THE IMAGE

The image that a client has of the Theta practitioner is an important part of a reading. As a practitioner, you must assume a *persona* of relative enlightenment. It is your responsibility to help people get closer to the divine, not to break their bubble. You don't have the luxury of letting clients see into your emotional life. They have certain expectations and it is your responsibility to do your best to live up to those expectations. Here are several pointers:

- Don't become emotionally wrapped up in a client's drama/trauma. It is not good for you to have an emotional meltdown in front of a client! This will also block you from witnessing the healing.

- Ask the Creator if a client can safely be a close friend before you make them one.

- There will be times when a client comes in for a reading, only to become emotional. They may even end up yelling at you. This can quickly put you off-balance and nine times out of ten, it will have nothing to do with you.

- As a healer, you have the challenge of staying in a good space under the most adverse of conditions. Never let the client see you sweat. At the end of day you should be back in your body, grounded, cleansed of negativity and in a good mood. In order to take care of others, you have to first take care of yourself.

- Without even knowing it, you may be treating someone the way that their negative subconscious is projecting. In thought and deed, in spoken word and in action, we must all treat others with kindness. In order to do this, it is important to know the difference between our feelings, programmes and beliefs and those of another.

LISTENING TO THE DIVINE

It is important to develop the ability to listen 'past your ego'. Learn to hear how to heal someone, how to hear truth and how to hear the Creator's explanation.

Hearing someone's thoughts can be difficult, particularly if they are thinking that they hate your guts! But if you can say to yourself, 'I can love them anyway,' it makes a big difference, at least most of the time.

CONFIDENTIALITY

Keep things that are confidential as secret and sacred as possible. Do not name names or begin gossip. If you can see that someone is in danger, sometimes there won't be a lot you can do. In these situations, you have to let the Creator direct you.

SANCTIMONIOUSNESS

It can be a challenge to prevent your own ethics from becoming involved in a reading. I believe that when people share secrets such as 'I'm having an affair with so and so, it is not my place to see it as wrong. I go up and ask the Creator for the truth in the situation. My outside opinion would be that you are mistaken anytime you are hurting anyone, but I do not bring this opinion into a reading.

Truth, by the way, isn't blurting out and telling the client, 'I can see that you are having an affair,' because honouring another person's truth is also important. When I do readings I sometimes have people ask me questions so that I don't talk about things that they don't want me to find out about.

'WHY?'

As practitioners, we think we have to understand why something is the way it is in a reading. However, it is not necessary for us to get caught up in the emotional drama of a person's story. As a reader, understand that something just 'is', rather than ask *why* it is. As a healer, understand that the sickness 'is' and needs to be changed. If an emotional component is causing the disease, then a belief needs to be released or a feeling instilled. But do not become emotionally attached to the causes of the sickness.

For instance, if the emotional cause of the disease is related to pain from a cheating ex-wife or (ex-husband), there is no need for you to attempt to understand why the ex-wife or husband cheated, just know that they did. Simply change the programmes associated with the ex-wife or husband. Not everything or everyone is going to make sense to you as a healer.

TRUTH

In a reading, always ask for the highest truth. Just say to the Creator, 'Show me the highest truth.' If you go up to connect and the energy that you connect to has a feeling of chaos, fear or anger, it probably isn't pure truth. Highest truth has a calm feeling to it.

For instance, let's say you are in a dangerous part of town and you receive a message that calmly tells you, 'Time to leave!' If you feel clear and calm about the message, it is undeniable truth.

Truth is actually a funny thing. One truth is that there are terrible things in the world, and if you are going to be a good intuitive you are going to see the bad things as well as the good. When you begin to see the real truth about people, you may never want to work with anyone ever again! You may need instruction from the Creator on how to love a person in spite of what you see.

Everyone is a product of their genetics and what they have grown up with. *If you could see a person's complete and whole divine truth, you would not make as critical a judgement of them.*

If someone comes in for a reading and you can sense that they are unstable, you are in a difficult situation as regards seeing the truth about them. Do you turn them away? Do you speak your truth and tell them that you know? Or do you help them gently and calmly? Would that be wise? Are they dangerous? All these questions will enter into your mind. And of course the truth is that unstable people need help just like anyone else, as long as you are not in personal danger from them.

Once you begin to do this work and commune with the Creator you will also have to beware of the human ego – your own and that of others. Ego will not slip in if you know that it is the Creator who does the work and who permits you to witness the work. This takes some of the burden from you when a person comes to you and says, 'You are my last and only hope.' In this instance it is time to state to them, 'The Creator can make you well and I will pray for you.' This will keep your ego out of the process.

Explore yourself and see if you need the following feelings of truth:

'It is safe to see truth.'

'I understand what truth feels like.'

'I understand the truth of another person's reality.'

'I am able to discern the highest truth through the Creator of All That Is.'

DISCERNMENT OF TRUTH: WHERE ARE YOUR THOUGHTS COMING FROM?

People always assume that the Creator talks to me non-stop and I know what to do all the time. However, I still have random thoughts coming into my mind and I have to discern whether these are coming from the Creator or are just some other thought forms floating around.

What you should know is that the mind processes thousands of thoughts all the time. In fact, my husband, Guy, says it is not fair to fight about the *thoughts* of his that I can hear, because they are just random thoughts that go through his mind. It is true that you cancel certain thoughts even as they go through your mind and you don't act on most of your thoughts. This is why you have to be focused and sort out what is from the Creator and what is not … and this takes a little bit of practice. Another complication is that sometimes people start listening to different spirit guides, and guides have their own opinions.

You also have to decide if you are picking up people's thoughts when you are doing a reading. In some instances, you may pick up what their biggest fear is. The one thing that people do not realize is that there are no secrets in a reading, at least not with a good intuitive. I find it amusing when clients come for a reading then try to put up a guard. If they give you verbal consent and then try to block you, it only makes it easier to read their thoughts anyway.

There is actually no such thing as a secret in the universe. If you take this on board and then live your life knowing everyone in the world can see into your soul, it will definitely change the way you live. I think it has changed the way I live.

As a Theta practitioner, it is important to train the mind to be discerning. You must be sure that you are able to distinguish between what is coming from the Creator of All That Is and what is coming from other people, while not shutting out other important vibrations or going into mental overload.

The question to ask is always: 'Is this the Creator's truth?'

A good example of this was when my brother-in-law came to visit me. He had had problems with cancer and at the time it was getting worse. When he walked into the room, the first thought that came into my mind was, 'Oh, the cancer is everywhere!' This thought was not mine; it was emanating from *him.* But it hit me like a wave on the ocean and momentarily I went into absolute panic – at least until I went up and asked the Creator what the truth was. I was told the cancer was not 'everywhere' but localized in one place. This was later confirmed by my brother-in-law's doctors. I had picked up on his fear, not the truth.

THE CREATOR'S TRUTH

In a reading you will perceive a person's truth (the truth that they have created for themselves), but the Creator's truth may be different.

Many years ago, before I met Guy, I was in a relationship with a person I wasn't compatible with. I stayed with them because I was afraid of change, and because the situation was potentially volatile, I was hesitant to make a definite end to the relationship.

During this time, I had conversations with God. My truth about the situation and the Creator's were always different. The Creator's truth was: 'This person came into your life and you allowed them to walk all over you. You are still allowing them to take advantage of you. You could have said "no" or dealt with the situation in many ways, but in reality, Vianna, you allowed this to happen. It was such good drama.'

Admitting to myself that I wasn't happy and wanted change was more than I could handle at the time. I just couldn't do it and I made excuses for the situation. Nevertheless, the Creator's truth was: 'Have you finished with this yet? Do you want to change? Would you like to know how? You need to release yourself from any obligations to this person. Change your belief systems and this person will fade away from your life.'

To be honest, I didn't know how to let myself be loved in any of my relationships before I met Guy. I was smart enough to leave those relationships, but I also had a definite programme that I *had* to leave them before I found my man from Montana. Maybe I chose people that I knew I could walk away from. When I got together with Guy, I could actually see myself sitting in a rocking chair and growing old with him. I had finally found someone that I could envision myself being with for the rest of my life. And the belief work formed right when I met him.

I believe that as we develop, we come together with our soul families with divine timing.

I believe that part of our divine truth is coming together with those families and working on our belief systems.

I believe that we are here to connect to the Creator's energy and *to learn*. This is the really important thing – to learn something wonderful from this existence. I have learned many wonderful things from the different people in my life.

If you are having difficulties in your marriage or relationship, energy test yourself for these programmes:

'It is OK to be loved.'

'I know it is safe to be loved.'

'I know what it feels like to be happy.'

'It is wrong to be happy.'

'It is selfish to be happy.'

'If I am happy, something bad will happen.'

'If I become close to someone, they will hurt me.'

As you become aware of these negative programmes, remember that some of them have helped you to survive and even thrive. Don't let yourself become overwhelmed and say, 'I have so much *stuff* to work on.' Instead, think, 'I have a lot to work on, but I know that when I have finished I will be a better person. I will understand why I have the belief systems that I do and I will know how to change them.'

THE PROJECTION OF BELIEFS

One of the most important things to avoid in readings is projecting your beliefs onto others. For instance, if you are having problems with your spouse, you may be so emotionally unbalanced by your own situation that you may think that *everybody* is having problems in their relationship.

I learned how easy this sort of thing can be from a young man who gave readings in my office. He was gay and began to tell many of the people that he was giving readings to that they were also gay. He was so much in his own world that he wanted everyone to be like him. He set out on a one-man quest to tell everyone that they were inherently attracted to the same sex.

I was first alerted by his behaviour when one of his clients spilled the beans. She had been married for 28 years, but told me that everything was going to fall apart in her life because she had just found out that she was gay. I asked her why she thought this and she told me that the young man had told her in a reading that she was definitely gay, there was no doubt about it.

I was stunned that someone could put such an untruth into a reading. I asked her, 'Do you love your husband?'

She answered, 'Of course I love my husband.'

'Do you enjoy having sex with your husband?'

'Yes, I enjoy having sex with my husband.'

'Well then, you're not gay, so stop worrying about it.'

After that I had to do a little more damage control with some of the other people whom the young man had given readings to. He became such a nuisance that I had to ask him to leave.

This is why you must be extremely careful in a reading. People can be so vulnerable when they come for intuitive advice that sometimes they will give you control of their life. It is so important that when you tell someone about their future, you tell them that *they* are creating that future, because people will sometimes create what you tell them.

Let us say you are deep into a reading with a client. Suddenly, you have one of those psychic epiphanies and tell the person, 'Oh, you're not getting along with your sweetheart.'

Since you have seen this far into their life, it has become your job to help them resolve their issue and perhaps help them rebuild their relationship. At this juncture in the reading you must be very careful with the client. They may be poised to break up with their lover and will blame you.

The situation may have come about because they are not able to feel another's love or concern or they feel they may never be able to please their sweetheart as a spouse. The issue with the relationship may not have anything at all to do with the other person, but everything to do with feelings that the client themselves lacks.

It is also very important for you as a reader to avoid projecting any of your own emotions into the situation, *particularly if you are having relationship problems of your own*. This is where the belief and feeling work come into the reading. The client should be given the choice to accept or deny the feeling of 'I know how to receive love'. At the same time, if you do belief work with them, they may come to the realization that they want to reconnect with their spouse. This is their choice. Your job is to help them become emotionally stable and able to make proper decisions for themselves.

THE PROJECTION OF PERCEPTION

In thought and deed, in spoken word and action, we must treat others with kindness. In order to do this, it is important to intuitively know the difference between our feelings, programmes and beliefs and those of another person.

Programmes we were taught as children such as 'Oh, get away from me!' can become projections of who we are in the here and now. This is to say we may project these programmes outwardly with thought forms that can manifest themselves on all levels: spiritually, physically, mentally and emotionally. Then, in some instances, other people will treat us according to what we are projecting.

The way that you perceive and project yourself on a conscious level is not necessarily what you are projecting subconsciously and psychically. You may think you are fine but still have programmes that were accepted as a child floating inside your unconscious mind. These programmes can cause disruption in the way you are interacting with other people and the way they are interacting with you.

In a reading, therefore, it is important to be wary of projected thought forms from the client. Without even knowing it, you may end up treating someone the way that their negative subconscious is projecting.

The goal, obviously, is for us all to have Seventh-Plane interaction with one another. This kind of interaction would raise us above competition, hatred and jealousy, not to mention all of the lesser base emotions that block us from being all that we can be with others as well as ourselves.

We must learn to *interact* instead of *reacting* in our relationships with people. If we can do this, through changing the way we intuitively perceive and send out messages, we can change the world.

Perception of information is also an important factor in the understanding of sacred knowledge. Many factors come into play here, including the background of the intuitive, their present state of mind and their physical state, as well as their spiritual development. These all affect their ability to listen to and discern sacred knowledge. An intuitive must learn to fine-tune their perceptions so that they can find the essence of acceptance without the interference of negative, or even positive, influences that can block development.

CONSCIOUS ACCEPTANCE

Let me be clear on another aspect of a reading. In a belief work session, you cannot ask the client if they will permit you to download multiple feelings and belief programmes for them; you have to get their verbal permission for each programme and belief in turn. If you connect to the Creator and find a feeling that the Creator tells you the person could benefit from, it is still your responsibility to tell that person what the feeling is so that they can consciously accept or refuse this energy. You may even go so far as to ask the Creator the possible ramifications should the person accept the feeling.

Belief programmes and feelings are not toys to play with and then discard as we please. These essences from the Creator are life-changing forces that will change a person's vibration and should not be taken lightly, either by the practitioner or by the client. For a practitioner to arrogantly think that they know what beliefs and programmes another person needs and then attempt to download these essences into them without verbal permission is the personification of conceit.

In this case, it is also unlikely that the person's unconscious mind will accept these energies, because it is hardwired to protect itself from programmes that it is currently unfamiliar with. Most outside influences, such as downloads and thought forms, that are not consciously accepted are automatically rejected by the unconscious mind in what might be termed a 'autonomic survival reflex'. This reflex is designed to protect us from the negative thoughts and emotions of others and enable us to tell the difference between our own thoughts and those of another person. In some people, it works so well that they are never affected by the thoughts of others. People who are intuitive, on the other hand, must develop the ability to understand all the information that is coming to them from the thoughts of others as well as other 'metaphysical' energies.

Regardless, each one of us needs to make the conscious choice whether or not to accept any programmes and feelings, whatever another person may think. For instance, I might know with every fibre of my being that my husband needs the belief programme of 'I know how to express myself' on every level. According to the Sixth-Plane Law of Free Will, though, I cannot download it into him while I am in another room and expect him to accept

21

it on every level of his being. His unconscious mind is hardwired to reject such thought forms. Similarly, a Theta practitioner cannot place their hand on a book of downloads and place the other hand on a person's shoulder and ask them if they would like to accept all the programmes in the book. The unconscious mind does not work like this. This is because of the *Law of Free Will.*

FREE WILL AND FREE AGENCY

Free will and free agency are beliefs that humans have the power to make their own choices. The spiritual connotations of free agency give the individual the self-authority to connect to what they perceive as God or the Creator. In ThetaHealing, we have the free agency to connect to the inner and outer aspects of the divine within ourselves as well as outside ourselves.

While we are given the tools of *morals* and *respect* for others, we have free will as to whether or not to put these into use. The Creator loves us enough to allow us our own opportunities to experience the joy of life without interference. As we move through this existence, we are given opportunities to create some of our own pathways to find our way. Our existence here can be perceived as a beautiful learning process of physical, mental and spiritual exploration.

Free will has been considered important to moral judgement by many religious authorities – and also criticized as a form of individualist ideology. The principle has religious, ethical, psychological and scientific implications. For example, in religion free will may imply that God does not assert power over individual will and choices. In ethics it may imply that an individual can be held accountable for their actions. In psychology it may imply that the mind controls at least some of the actions of the body. In the scientific realm, it may imply that the actions of the body, including the brain, are not wholly determined by physical causality. (Causality is the principle of cause and effect.)[1]

The concept of free will was first brought to the forefront of controversy in the fourth century by a British priest called Pelagius. His writings did not survive the ages, but one of his disciples wrote down some of what he believed. These beliefs were diametrically opposed to those held by the Church and St Augustine. Since that time, the issue of free will has continued to be a question on the minds of spiritual, religious and even scientific thinkers.

One view is that humanity has the capacity to seek God quite apart from any movement of God's Word or the Holy Spirit. We don't have complete

---

Resource: Wikipekia.

control over all things, but can co-operate with God to a certain degree in this salvation effort: we can (unaided by grace) make the first move toward God, and God will then complete the salvation process. This teaching is the doctrine of *synergeia*, or *synergy*, in that the process of salvation is co-operation between God and humanity from start to finish.

Whatever our views may be, free will is an enduring principle. As it relates to our abilities, as it pertains to the divine, to individuals in the grand scheme of things, even to the brain controlling the body, it will simply not be extinguished. There have been many attempts to override it through the ages and even in ThetaHealing some people have attempted to download programmes and beliefs into people without their *conscious acceptance*. As already explained, while these divine thought forms may be sent with the best of intentions, they will never be effective unless the person consciously accepts them.

Always remember: free agency and free will are important branches on the tree of ThetaHealing.

4

ADVANCED HEALING

There are generally four ways to do energy healing:

- through the *chi* energy of the body
- through the electrical energy of the mind
- through spiritual energies that are brought in
- through the Creator of All That Is.

All these ways of healing are of the Creator, but the latter is the simplest.

WITNESS THE CREATOR HEAL

Sometimes we use the electrical energy of the mind to create changes in the body. If you are using your mind to heal, however, you are likely to be tired when you have finished. If you witness the Creator doing the healing, on the other hand, you will feel awake and alive once you have finished. Witnessing the Creator heal also keeps the ego out of the healing. You should be patient and wait for the Creator's energy to come in, then simply *witness* it instead of trying to *force* it with your own energy.

A good example of a *forced healing* using the mind was in a session I had with a woman who came in with a melanoma on her face. Melanoma is a very dangerous type of cancer and, if left untreated, can quickly spread through the body. I was very concerned and annoyed with the woman for letting the disease advance as far as it had. All I could think was, 'Why did you let it go this far without going to the doctor?!' This was years ago, before I was taught extra patience by the Creator. I went up and asked for the melanoma to be gone from her body *now* and *pushed* the healing through with my mind, using the energy of my annoyance and imagining it being gone from her skin.

Instead of just watching it happen through the Creator, I imagined reaching in and taking it out.

She came in the next day with a big hole in her face – it seems the cancerous growth had inexplicably fallen out. Eventually, the hole filled up perfectly, but the Creator would have undoubtedly healed the skin as the cancer was removed without leaving a gaping hole.

What I learned from this was: *don't force the healing!*

In total, it took me seven years to finally learn to let go and say 'Creator, show me what needs to be done' instead of trying to add my two bits. Eventually I realized that even though I understand much of what goes on in the body, I do not have the Creator's understanding of disease. In a healing, I might have an overview of what needs to be done, but on an all-encompassing level, I do not understand things as the Creator does. By the time I have figured out all that needs to be done on a molecular or even on a subatomic level, I might well have been in the body for 50 years trying to work out the who, what, where and why of the healing. And all this is ego.

So I strongly suggest that you simply ask the Creator to show you what needs to be done for the healing to work as it should. Just say, 'Creator, do what needs to be done. Show me.' You don't have to completely understand the disorder; you just have to witness it healed.

The more I read credible scientific journals, the more I realize how easy it is to change molecular structure. And if the Creator knows how to make it the way that it is, then the Creator knows how to fix it, and I can ask for an explanation later.

FUSING THE HEALER AND THE PSYCHIC

ThetaHealing is designed to open up your *psychic abilities to heal*. Most people do not realize that being psychic and being a healer are two different skills. Putting the two together is the key.

Both bring their pressures. The *healer* is expected to witness the condition healed and the *body psychic* is expected to see inside the body.

Accordingly, as a psychic, you should practise seeing and recognizing different viruses, bacteria, parasites and heavy metals, so you know what they look and feel like in the body. The client will expect you to identify these influences with accuracy.

As a healer, you are put on the spot in a different way. You do not have to know what the disease is to have the Creator heal it – you only need to know that a person has something wrong – but you have to put yourself in a deep enough meditative state to witness it changed, to witness the healing *done*.

There are 'high' and 'low' Theta states that people use in ThetaHealing. The 'high' is not as effective as the 'low' in major healing. Be sure to take your time to be in a deep Theta state when you facilitate a healing.

A ThetaHealer is a combination of healer and psychic: a healer who uses their psychic abilities to witness a healing through a connection to the Creator.

THE HEALING PROCESS

FEELING HEALTHY

When a person comes to me for a healing, one of the first things I do is have the Creator teach them what it feels like to be healthy, because some people don't know what that feels like. From that point on in the session, they will immediately feel better and it is much more likely that they will accept a physical healing.

The following is the step-by-step healing process:

THE COMPLETE PROCESS FOR HEALING AND GROUNDING

1. Centre yourself in your heart and visualize yourself going down into Mother Earth, which is part of All That Is.

2. Visualize bringing up the energy through your feet, opening up all of your chakras as you go. Continue going up out of your crown chakra, in a beautiful ball of light, out to the universe.

3. Go beyond the universe, past the white lights, past the dark light, past the white light, past the jelly-like substance that is the Laws, into a pearly iridescent white light, into the Seventh Plane of Existence.

4. Gather unconditional love and make the command: *'Creator, it is commanded that this person be healed now. Thank you. It is done. It is done. It is done.'*

5. Witness the healing energy going into the person's space and watch the changes and shifts being made. Continue to watch until they are completed.

6. Imagine rinsing yourself off with a stream of water or white light.

7. To ground yourself properly, imagine your energy coming back into your space then going into the Earth, and then pull it up through all your chakras to your crown chakra. As you become used to this practice, it will no longer be necessary to ground back into your body because of the realization that you are not really separate but a part of All That Is.

8. Perform a physical energy break (as outlined in *ThetaHealing*). This will keep your body balanced.

UNCONDITIONAL LOVE

In order to make a molecular change in the body, one must have energy to create or 'dis-create'. Where does this energy come from in a healing?

When you go up to the Creator of All That Is for a healing, you reach up and grab the energy of *unconditional love* and put it in the body. This enables the body to have the energy it needs to make changes. It only takes one atom of unconditional love to make any change in the body.

In beginners' classes, we teach students a step-by-step process to visualize 'going up' and gathering the love. As the brain gets used to what it is supposed to be visualizing, the process will happen spontaneously and automatically.

In the end it is the ability of the practitioner to *witness* the healing that will bring it into being. The Creator does the healing, the practitioner witnesses it and there it is. There is a law in physics that says nothing exists unless it is witnessed.

In ThetaHealing classes, the group healing process teaches people to accept unconditional love from the Creator and introduces the groups to the belief and feeling work. However, if you force unconditional love into the body of a person who has never received it, their body will fight it off, just as it would a bacteria or virus. The person themselves will become uncomfortable and feel out of sorts with the whole thing. The practitioner will be able to sense this rejection. This is the time to energy test the person for the programme of 'I can accept unconditional love'. If they indicate that they do not know how to accept unconditional love, they give their permission and the practitioner instills the feeling from the Creator.

To have *unconditional love* for people is to love them in a 'Christ' or 'Buddha' consciousness. This is to see their truth through the Creator (or with enlightenment) and still love them in spite of it.

It has been my experience that programmes associated with the acceptance of unconditional love are generally created in childhood. For instance, a mother might show real love to her child only to beat it mercilessly immediately after. Or in another scenario, a father might express real love to a child and then molest it. Childhood situations such as this create programmes that mean the person doesn't know how to receive unconditional love.

I have also observed that some survivors of severe child abuse are able to anticipate what a person is going to do before they do it. For obvious reasons, this survival reflex has made them very psychic. I think that many children of abuse have developed the same way. To get out of their own space and intuitively watch others is natural for them because they are used to it. These kinds of people have focused on being in other people's space for most of their early life. They are looking for love.

To a large extent, all our lives are filled with the search for love in all its shapes and forms. To find examples, we need only to observe the driving force to find a soul mate, to have friends, to bear and raise children, to have pets, and so on. Men have competitive sports events to feel comradely and to bond with one another. Even some anger and hatred is the result of the search for love, or the loss or lack of love. Most human relations of a positive nature are a search for the essence of love.

A large number of the people you work with will be searching in vain for love and will not be able to find it no matter how hard they look. This may be because they don't love themselves and they don't understand what it feels like to love. With permission, instill the feeling of pure love into them on all levels from the Creator.

INSTANT HEALING

Some people need to be healed more than once due to the nature of the difficulties they are experiencing. These may be spiritual, mental, physical or emotional. Other people are ready to be healed instantly and completely.

If the body does not receive an instant healing when given the command, there is a subconscious programme blocking it. This programme must be found and changed. People who have no blocks to stop the healing will heal instantly.

Other people who come to you will not believe they can be healed and will need downloads in order to change. As long as you don't become discouraged, the Creator will assist you in finding the appropriate feeling, emotion or belief, as will the person themselves. The mind, body and spirit of a person all have a memory like a computer and if you know the right questions to ask, these aspects will tell you what needs to be released and replaced or what feeling is missing.

It is possible, however, that you will misinterpret these messages and become discouraged. Perhaps this feeling is not your own, but is being projected from the person that is being healed. Perhaps they do not know how to live without being discouraged and have lost hope.

It is my belief that there are only a few essential feelings and beliefs for every healing. It is my understanding that disease is developed by having certain beliefs over a long period of time. Once these beliefs are cleared, the sickness leaves. It was there to get your attention, to tell you that something was out of synch, out of focus or out of balance with the body.

The goal is to clear the body, mind and soul of enough burdening beliefs to have pure and unadulterated communication with the Creator. So it is also my belief that ThetaHealing is not just about clearing disease but about enabling humanity to communicate with the Creator of All That Is.

HEALING WITH CHILDREN

The chances of a successful healing with a child are very high. Children have a pure conviction in the reality of the divine and generally will not block or hinder a healing. However, parents are often locked into their child's problem so deeply that they will not permit the child to heal. They may have created beliefs that the child is and always will be sick and that nothing can help them. This interferes with the healing process.

So, with children, you should work with the parents' belief systems. The biggest challenge is to get them to realize that their child can change. Work with the belief systems of both parents, especially the mother. Both parents need encouragement to know that the child can and will get better.

Love is the key element in healing a child. *Check to see if they believe they have to be ill to get their parents' attention.* If they are old enough, ask for permission to heal them. 'Old enough' means that they are able to speak.

In certain instances, children heal but are then put back into the environment that made them sick. Pollution, heavy metals, poor diet and lack of nurturing can all be factors.

Once, in a class consisting of little children, I guided the whole group up into Theta. Then I had the little tykes do body scans on one another. Time and again they would correctly report what they experienced while doing readings. These children could learn in four hours what it takes adults three days to learn.

One of the reasons for this was that they still had the 'I think I can' energy. Ask yourself, would you like to know what the 'I think I can' energy *feels like* again? This is a childhood programme that many of us lose along the way.

Would you like to know that everything that you've done up to this point in your life actually *matters*?

I like this saying: 'Childhood is supposed to be a great part of life, but we seem to spend most of our lives getting over it.' Beginnings can be hard and endings are sad, but it's the middle that counts. If life is hard, give time for hope to float (from the movie *Hope Floats*).

BELIEFS AND ILLNESS

I believe that in some instances people draw viruses and bacteria to them because of beliefs associated with the fear of them.

We all know people in our day-to-day lives who hardly ever fall ill and people who are more prone to it. You might say that some people have better immune systems. I think that the reason they have superior immune systems is that they believe that they do. For instance, some people believe that if they walk barefoot in the snow they are going to get a cold. Others think that little children are breeding grounds for sickness. Still others believe that they cannot be around a certain illness or they will catch it.

If these beliefs were true for everyone, doctors, nurses and teachers would be ill all the time. Why can nurses be around sick people and usually not become sick themselves? It is because they don't have the pervading fear of disease. If we didn't have these fearless people in the world, no one would work with people who had infectious diseases because we would all be too terrified of catching them.

VIRUSES AND BELIEFS

We pick our diseases the way we pick our mates: we are drawn to each other because of our matching vibrations and belief systems. When we have the same belief system as a virus, bacterium, yeast or fungus, a weakness is created in our immune system. The virus, bacterium, yeast or fungus is then drawn to us and is able to attach to us.

I know this is a bold statement, but I came to this conclusion through working with a woman with genital herpes. As I explained in *ThetaHealing*, I worked with her for a very long time, but the herpes wouldn't go away. Eventually the Creator told me to change the belief systems on the *virus* as well as on her. So I started pulling belief systems around it and as I pulled the bottom belief systems, I watched it change into something completely different and leave the body. It was gone, and this was confirmed by doctors.

What is really happening during this process, in scientific terms? It is a scientific theory that bacteria will become a virus and a virus will become a fungus and will actually evolve into something different again, thus escaping detection. When belief work is done on a virus, it changes again, but this time into a harmless form of energy. Understand, we are not *killing* the virus; rather we are *transforming* it by witnessing the rearrangement of its subatomic particles. Everything can be changed in the body if you witness the rearrangement of the subatomic particles.

5

THE CREATION OF FEELINGS

Some people have never experienced the energy of certain feelings in their lives. Perhaps they were traumatized as a child and did not develop these feelings, or lost them somewhere in the drama of this existence. But in order to bring, for example, joy or love into our lives, we have to *experience* them first. We have to be shown what they feel like by the Creator. The Advanced ThetaHealing class was developed to give people a set of 'feeling downloads'.

The speeds at which changes are made with feeling work are amazing. What might take people lifetimes to learn can be learned in seconds. People can be taught quickly what it *feels like* to be loved, honoured, respected, cherished, even to live *without* a negative feeling created by habit. An example of this would be 'I know how to live without being miserable'.

As I explained in *ThetaHealing*, as with belief work, with feeling work the practitioner energy tests the client (or themselves) to find if they have or have or have not experienced specific feelings. They then get the client's verbal permission and connect with the Creator of All That Is. Using the command process, they witness the energy of the feeling downloads from the Creator flowing through every cell of the person's body on all four belief levels. Once this feeling has been experienced, the person is ready to create life changes.

I believe that by using the feeling work we are actually training our cells how to live without certain feelings, such as depression. The feeling work gives us the ability to literally change our mind, to reset the receptors for depression or other unwanted feelings and to open new receptors that can be created when in a Theta wave.

You may ask, 'What is the proof for this?' I offer the evidence that many people start to get well when they begin to use the feeling work. For instance, simply instilling what it *feels like* to live without being defeated can bring about positive changes in diabetes and help other diseases as well.

Feelings are downloaded from the Creator of All That Is in the following process:

THE CREATION OF FEELINGS PROCESS

1. Centre yourself. Begin by sending your consciousness down into the centre of Mother Earth, which is part of All That Is. Bring the energy up through your feet, into your body and up through all the chakras.

2. Go beyond the universe, past the white lights, past the dark light, past the white light, past the jelly-like substance that is the Laws, into a pearly iridescent white light, into the Seventh Plane of Existence.

3. Connect with the Creator of All That Is and make the following command: *'Creator of All That Is, it is commanded to instill the feeling of* [name the feeling] *into* [name the person] *through every cell of their body, on all four belief levels and in every area of their life, in the highest and best way. Thank you. It is done. It is done. It is done.'*

4. Witness the energy of the feeling flow into the person's space and visualize the feeling from the Creator moving through every cell of the person's body, instilling the feeling on all four belief levels.

5. When you have finished, move your consciousness out of the person's space through the crown chakra and disconnect by rinsing yourself off in a stream of water or white light. Enter your body through your crown chakra, send your consciousness down into Mother Earth, then pull the energy up through your body to the top of your crown and perform an energy break.

In time, as you become more comfortable with this process, grounding will not be necessary.

DOWNLOADS

There are variations of feelings and knowledge that a person may have never experienced. When these are downloaded into them, they attain an awareness that is integrated into their All That Is by the Creator of All That Is of the Seventh Plane of Existence. Teaching these feelings will have a dramatic effect upon the abilities of the intuitive person and will create physical well-being and greater spiritual awareness.

It is important to consider downloading the feelings listed here, both for yourself and others. Then everything that doesn't serve can be easily released.

The more that you clear your mind in this way, the more you can access the Seventh Plane easily to bring the body to balance. Illness is not your enemy. Disease is merely a sign of imbalance.

❖❖❖❖❖

The following programmes and feelings are in these categories:

'I know the Creator's definition of...'

'I know what it feels like to...'

'I know what it feels like to understand how to...'

'I know when...'

'I know how...'

'I know how to live my daily life and...'

'I know the Creator's perspective on...'

'I know it is possible to...'

Here are some examples:

'I know *the Creator's definition of trust.*'

'I know *what it feels like to trust.*'

'I know *what it feels like to understand how to trust.*'

'I know *when to trust.*'

'I know *how to trust.*'

'I know *how to live my daily life and trust.*'

'I know *the Creator's perspective on trust.*'

'I know *it is possible to trust.*'

Even though I am giving you the following downloads here, it would still be worthwhile attending an Advanced ThetaHealing class with a certified instructor.

Programmes of the Creator of All That Is

'I understand what it feels like to be totally connected to the Creator of All That Is.'

'I know how to be totally connected to the Creator of All That Is.'

'I know the Creator of All That Is.'

'I understand what it feels like to allow the Creator to show me the inside of the body.'

'I know how to allow the Creator of All That Is to show me what is in the body.'

'I understand what it feels like to trust that the Creator will tell me exactly what I'm looking at in the body.'

'I know how to trust that the Creator will tell me exactly what I'm looking at in the body.'

'I know the difference between listening to the Creator of All That Is and myself.'

'I understand what it feels like to show others they are important to the Creator of All That Is.'

'I know how to show others they are important to the Creator of All That Is.'

'I understand what it feels like to radiate the energy of the Creator of All That Is to the world.'

'I know how to radiate the energy of the Creator of All That Is to the world.'

'I understand what it feels like to know the difference between listening to the Creator and to myself.'

'I understand what it feels like to be worthy of the love of the Creator of All That Is.'

'I understand what it feels like to know all things are possible with the Creator.'

'I understand what it feels like to know the Creator of All That Is.'

'I know it is possible to know that the Creator of All That Is exists.'

'I understand what it feels like to deserve the love of the Creator of All That Is.'

'I know that I deserve the love of the Creator of All That Is.'

'I understand what it feels like to connect to the Creator of All That Is.'

'I know how to connect to the Creator of All That Is.'

'I know the Creator of All That Is is totally connected to me.'

'I know how to live my daily life totally connected to the Creator of All That Is.'

'I understand what it feels like to witness the Creator of All That Is doing a healing.'

'I know how to witness the Creator of All That Is doing a healing.'

'I know when to witness the Creator of All That Is doing a healing.'

'I know how to live without feeling separate from the Creator of All That Is.'

Abundance

'I understand the Creator's definition of abundance.'

'I understand what it feels like to have abundance.'

'I know how to have abundance.'

'I know how to live my daily life with abundance.'

'I know the Creator's perspective on abundance.'

'I know it is possible to have abundance.'

Acceptance

'I understand the Creator's definition of acceptance.'

'I understand what acceptance feels like.'

'I know when to accept things.'

'I know how to accept things.'

'I know how to live my daily life with acceptance.'

'I know the Creator's perspective on acceptance.'

'I know it is possible to accept myself fully.'

'I understand what it feels like to accept and receive healing from another.'

'I know how to accept and receive healing from another.'

'I know the Creator's perspective on healing.'

'I know it is possible to accept and receive healing from another.'

Acceptance by the Creator

'I understand the Creator's definition of being completely accepted by the Creator of All That Is.'

'I understand what it feels like to be completely accepted by the Creator.'

'I know how to be completely accepted by the Creator.'

'I know how to live my daily life completely accepted by the Creator.'

'I know the Creator's perspective on being completely accepted by the Creator of All That Is.'

'I know it is possible to be completely accepted by the Creator.'

Accountability

'I understand the Creator's definition of accountability.'

'I understand what it feels like to be accountable.'

'I know when to be accountable.'

'I know how to be accountable.'

'I know how to live my daily life with accountability.'

'I know the Creator's perspective on accountability.'

'I know it is possible to be accountable for my own actions.'

Achievement

'I understand the Creator's definition of achievement.'

'I understand what it feels like to achieve.'

'I know when to achieve.'

'I know how to achieve.'

'I know how to live my daily life achieving.'

'I know the Creator's perspective on achievement.'

Articulating Feelings

'I understand the Creator's definition of articulating my feelings.'

'I understand what it feels like to articulate my feelings.'

'I know when to articulate my feelings.'

'I know how to articulate my feelings.'

'I know how to live my daily life articulating my feelings.'

'I know the Creator's perspective on articulating my feelings.'

'I know it is possible to articulate my feelings.'

Balance

'I understand the Creator's definition of balance.'

'I understand what it feels like to be balanced.'

'I know how to be balanced.'

'I know how to live my daily life in balance.'

'I know the Creator's perspective on balance.'

'I know it is possible to be balanced.'

Beauty

'I understand the Creator's definition of beauty.'

'I understand what it feels like to be beautiful.'

'I know how to live my daily life in beauty.'

'I know the Creator's perspective on beauty.'

'I know it is possible to be beautiful.'

Being Cherished

'I understand the Creator's definition of being cherished.'

'I understand what it feels like to be cherished.'

'I know how to be cherished.'

'I know how to live my daily life cherished by others.'

'I know the Creator's perspective on being cherished.'

'I know it is possible to be cherished.'

Being Complete

'I understand the Creator's definition of being complete.'

'I understand what it feels like to be complete.'

'I know how to be complete.'

'I know it is possible to be complete.'

Being Emotionally Present

'I understand the Creator's definition of being emotionally present.'

'I understand what it feels like to be emotionally present.'

'I know how to be emotionally present.'

'I know how to live my daily life emotionally present.'

'I know the Creator's perspective on being emotionally present.'

'I know it is possible to be emotionally present.'

Being Happy for Others

'I understand the Creator's definition of being happy for others.'

'I understand what it feels like to be happy for others.'

'I know when to be happy for others.'

'I know how to be happy for others.'

'I know how to live my daily life happy for others.'

'I know the Creator's perspective on being happy for others.'

'I know it is possible to be happy for others.'

Being Heard by Others

'I understand the Creator's definition of being heard by others.'

'I understand what it feels like to be heard by others.'

'I know when to be heard by others.'

'I know how to be heard by others.'

'I know how to live my daily life heard by others.'

'I know the Creator's perspective on being heard by others.'

'I know it is possible to be heard by others.'

Being in the Moment

'I understand the Creator's definition of being in the moment.'

'I understand what it feels like to be in the moment.'

'I know how to be in the moment.'

'I know how to live my daily life in the moment.'

'I know the Creator's perspective on being in the moment.'

'I know it is possible to be in the moment.'

'I understand what it feels like to live in the now, in this moment and this second.'

'I know how to live in the now, in this moment and this second.'

'I understand what it feels like to live in the now, experiencing the joy of it.'

Being Lovable

'I understand the Creator's definition of being loveable.'

'I understand what it feels like to be lovable.'

'I know how to be lovable.'

'I know the Creator's perspective on being lovable.'

'I know it is possible to be lovable.'

Being Loved by a Companion

'I understand the Creator's definition of being loved by my companion.'

'I understand what it feels like to be loved by my companion.'

'I know when to be loved by my companion.'

'I know how to be loved by my companion.'

'I know how to live my daily life loved by my companion.'

'I know the Creator's perspective on being loved by my companion.'

'I know it is possible to be loved by my companion.'

Being Open to Ideas

'I understand the Creator's definition of being open to ideas.'

'I understand what it feels like to be open to ideas.'

'I know when to be open to ideas.'

'I know how to be open to ideas.'

'I know how to live my daily life open to ideas.'

'I know it is possible to be open to all ideas.'

Being Special

'I understand what it feels like to be special.'

'I know how to be special.'

'I know the Creator's perspective on being special.'

'I know it is possible to be special.'

Being Understood by Others

'I understand the Creator's definition of being understood by others.'

'I understand what it feels like to be understood by others.'

'I know when to be understood by others.'

'I know how to be understood by others.'

'I know how to live my daily life understood by others.'

'I know the Creator's perspective on being understood by others.'

'I know it is possible to be understood by others.'

Being Wanted

'I understand the definition of being wanted through the Creator of All That Is.'

'I understand what it feels like to be wanted.'

'I know when to be wanted.'

'I know how to be wanted.'

'I know it is possible to be wanted.'

Being Whole

'I understand what it feels like to be whole.'

'I know how to be whole.'

'I know it is possible to be whole.'

Benevolence

'I understand the Creator's definition of benevolence.'

'I understand what it feels like to be benevolent.'

'I know true benevolence.'

'I know when to be benevolent.'

'I know how to be benevolent.'

'I know how to live my daily life benevolently.'

'I know the Creator's perspective on benevolence.'

'I know it is possible to be benevolent.'

The Breath of Life

'I understand the Creator's definition of the breath of life.'

'I understand what it feels like to receive the breath of life.'

'I know how to receive the breath of life.'

'I know how to live my daily life breathing in the breath of life.'

'I know the Creator's perspective on the breath of life.'

'I know it is possible to breathe.'

Calm

'I understand the Creator's definition of calm.'

'I understand what it feels like to be calm.'

'I know when to be calm.'

'I know how to be calm.'

'I know how to live my daily life calmly.'

'I know the Creator's perspective on being calm.'

'I know it is possible to be calm.'

Clairvoyance

'I understand the Creator's definition of seeing clairvoyantly.'

'I understand what it feels like to see clairvoyantly.'

'I know when to see clairvoyantly.'

'I know how to see clairvoyantly.'

'I know how to live my daily life seeing clairvoyantly.'

'I know the Creator's perspective on clairvoyance.'

'I know it is possible to see clairvoyantly.'

Clear Communication

'I understand the Creator's definition of communicating clearly.'

'I understand what it feels like to be able to communicate clearly.'

'I know how to be able to communicate clearly.'

'I know how to live my daily life communicating clearly.'

'I know the Creator's perspective on being able to communicate clearly.'

'I know it is possible to be able to communicate clearly.'

Common Sense

'I understand the Creator's definition of common sense.'

'I understand what it feels like to have common sense.'

'I know when to have common sense.'

'I know how to have common sense.'

'I know how to live my daily life with common sense.'

'I know the Creator's perspective on common sense.'

'I know it is possible to have common sense.'

Compassion

'I understand the Creator's definition of compassion.'

'I understand what it feels like to have compassion for myself and others.'

'I know true compassion.'

'I know when to have compassion.'

'I know how to have compassion.'

'I know how to live my daily life with compassion.'

'I know the Creator's perspective on compassion.'

'I know it is possible to have compassion for myself and others.'

Confidence

'I understand the definition of confidence through the Creator of All That Is.'

'I understand what it feels like to be confident.'

'I know when to be confident.'

'I know how to be confident.'

'I know how to live my daily life confidently.'

'I know the Creator's perspective on confidence.'

'I know it is possible to be confident.'

Co-operation

'I understand the Creator's definition of co-operation.'

'I understand what it feels like to be co-operative.'

'I know what co-operation is.'

'I know when to be co-operative.'

'I know how to live my daily life co-operatively.'

Debt

    'I understand the Creator's definition of being debt free.'

    'I understand what it feels like to be debt free.'

    'I know how to be debt free.'

    'I know how to live my daily life debt free.'

    'I know it is possible to be debt free.'

Dedication

    'I understand the Creator's definition of dedication.'

    'I understand what it feels like to be dedicated.'

    'I know how to be dedicated.'

    'I know how to live my daily life with dedication.'

    'I know the Creator's perspective on dedication.'

    'I know it is possible to be dedicated.'

    'I understand the Creator's definition of dedication to the Creator.'

    'I understand what it feels like to be dedicated to the Creator.'

    'I know how to be dedicated to the Creator.'

    'I know how to live my daily life dedicated to the Creator.'

    'I know the Creator's perspective on dedication to the Creator.'

    'I know it is possible to be dedicated to the Creator.'

    'I understand the Creator's definition of being dedicated to my goals.'

    'I understand what it feels like to be dedicated to my goals.'

    'I know when to be dedicated to my goals.'

    'I know how to be dedicated to my goals.'

    'I know how to live my daily life dedicated to my goals.'

    'I know the Creator's perspective on being dedicated to my goals.'

    'I know it is possible to be dedicated to my goals.'

Deserving to Shine

'I understand the Creator's definition of deserving to shine.'

'I understand what it feels like to deserve to shine.'

'I know how to deserve to shine.'

'I know how to live my daily life shining.'

'I know the perspective of deserving to shine through the Creator of All That Is.'

Devotion

'I understand the Creator's definition of devotion.'

'I understand what it feels like to be devoted.'

'I know what devotion is.'

'I know how to live my daily life with devotion.'

'I know the Creator's perspective on devotion.'

'I know it is possible to be devoted.'

Diligence

'I understand the Creator's definition of diligence.'

'I understand what it feels like to be diligent.'

'I know how to live my daily life diligently.'

'I know the Creator's perspective on diligence.'

'I know it is possible to be diligent.'

Evaluation

'I understand the Creator's definition of evaluation.'

'I understand what it feels like to evaluate a situation with clarity.'

'I know when to evaluate a situation.'

'I know how to evaluate a situation.'

'I know the Creator's perspective on evaluation.'

'I know it is possible to evaluate a situation before acting.'

Faith

'I understand the Creator's definition of faith.'

'I understand what it feels like to have faith.'

'I know how to live my daily life with faith.'

'I know the Creator's perspective on faith.'

'I know it is possible to have faith.'

Family

'I understand the Creator's definition of family.'

'I understand what it feels like to have a family.'

'I know when to have a family.'

'I know how to have a family.'

'I know the Creator's perspective on family.'

'I know it is possible to have a family.'

Focus

'I understand the Creator's definition of focus.'

'I understand what it feels like to focus.'

'I know when to focus.'

'I know how to focus.'

'I know how to live my daily life focused.'

'I know the Creator's perspective on focus.'

'I know it is possible to focus.'

Forgiveness

'I understand the Creator's definition of forgiveness.'

'I understand what it feels like to forgive myself and others.'

'I know true forgiveness.'

'I know when to forgive.'

'I know how to forgive.'

'I know how to live my daily life with forgiveness.'

'I know the Creator's perspective on forgiveness.'

'I know it is possible to forgive myself and others.'

Fun

'I understand the Creator's definition of fun.'

'I understand what it feels like to have fun.'

'I know when to have fun.'

'I know how to have fun.'

'I know how to live my daily life having fun.'

'I know the Creator's perspective on fun.'

'I know it is possible to have fun.'

Gratitude

'I understand the Creator's definition of gratitude.'

'I understand what it feels like to be grateful to others and to God.'

'I know when to be grateful.'

'I know how to grateful.'

'I know how to live my daily life in gratitude.'

'I know the Creator's perspective on gratitude.'

'I know it is possible to be grateful.'

Health

'I understand the Creator's definition of health.'

'I understand what it feels like to be healthy.'

'I know when I am healthy.'

'I know how to be healthy.'

'I know how to live my daily life in health.'

'I know the Creator's perspective on health.'

'I know it is possible to be healthy.'

Home

'I understand the Creator's definition of home.'

'I understand what it feels like to have a home.'

'I know how to have a home.'

'I know the Creator's perspective on home.'

'I know it is possible to have a home.'

Honesty

'I understand the Creator's definition of honesty.'

'I understand what it feels like to be honest.'

'I know when to be honest.'

'I know how to be honest.'

'I know how to live my daily life honestly.'

'I know the Creator's perspective on honesty.'

'I know it is possible to be honest.'

'I understand the Creator's definition of being honest with myself.'

'I understand what it feels like to be honest with myself.'

'I know how to be honest with myself.'

'I know how to live my daily life being honest with myself.'

'I know the Creator's perspective on being honest with myself.'

'I know it is possible to be honest with myself.'

Honour

'I understand the Creator's definition of honour.'

'I understand what it feels like to be honourable.'

'I know when to be honourable.'

'I know how to be honourable.'

'I know how to live my daily life with honour.'

'I know the Creator's perspective on honour.'

'I know it is possible to be honourable.'

Humility

'I understand the Creator's definition of humility.'

'I understand what it feels like to be humble.'

'I know when to be humble.'

'I know how to be humble.'

'I know the Creator's perspective on humility.'

'I know it is possible to be humble.'

Imperviousness

'I understand the Creator's definition of being impervious to doubt.'

'I understand what it feels like to be impervious to doubt.'

'I know how to be impervious to doubt.'

'I know how to live my daily life impervious to doubt.'

'I know the Creator's perspective on being impervious to doubt.'

'I know it is possible to be impervious to doubt.'

'I understand the Creator's definition of being impervious to toxicity.'

'I understand what it feels like to be impervious to toxicity.'

'I know how to be impervious to toxicity.'

'I know how to live my daily life impervious to toxicity.'

'I know it is possible to be impervious to toxicity.'

'I understand the Creator's definition of being impervious to negativity.'

'I understand what it feels like to be impervious to negativity.'

'I know how be impervious to negativity.'

'I know how to live my daily life impervious to negativity.'

'I know it is possible to be impervious to negativity.'

'I understand the Creator's definition of being impervious to worry.'

'I understand what it feels like to be impervious to worry.'

'I know how to be impervious to worry.'

'I know how to live my daily life impervious to worry.'

'I know it is possible to be impervious to worry.'

'I understand the Creator's definition of being impervious to disease.'

'I understand what it feels like to be impervious to disease.'

'I know how to be impervious to disease.'

'I know how to life my daily life impervious to disease.'

'I know it is possible to be impervious to disease.'

Importance

'I understand the Creator's definition of importance.'

'I understand what it feels like to feel important.'

'I know how to live my daily life feeling important.'

'I know the Creator's perspective on importance.'

'I know it is possible to be important to the Creator of All That Is.'

Integrity

'I understand the Creator's definition of integrity.'

'I understand what it feels like to have integrity.'

'I know how to have integrity.'

'I know how to live my daily life with integrity.'

'I know the Creator's perspective on integrity.'

'I know it is possible to be full of integrity.'

Interaction with Others

'I understand the Creator's definition of interaction with others.'

'I understand what it feels like to interact with others.'

'I know when to interact with others.'

'I know how to interact with others.'

'I know how to live my daily life interacting with others.'

'I know it is possible to interact with others.'

Instant Healing

'I understand the Creator's definition of instant healing.'

'I understand what it feels like to witness instant healing.'

'I know how to witness instant healing.'

'I know the Creator's perspective on instant healing.'

'I know it is possible to witness instant healing.'

Intuition

'I understand the Creator's definition of true intuition.'

'I understand what it feels like to trust my intuition.'

'I know when to trust my intuition.'

'I know how to trust my intuition.'

'I know how to live my daily life trusting my intuition.'

'I know it is possible to trust my intuition.'

Joy

'I understand the Creator's definition of joy.'

'I understand what it feels like to be joyful.'

'I know how to be joyful.'

'I know how to live my daily life in joy.'

'I know the Creator's perspective on joy.'

'I know it is possible to be joyful.'

Knowing That the Creator Is Real

'I understand what it feels like to know that the Creator is real.'

'I know how to live my daily life knowing the Creator is real.'

'I know it is possible that the Creator is real.'

Knowing Your True Self

'I understand what it feels like to know my true self.'

'I know my true self.'

'I know the Creator's perspective on my true self.'

'Let It Be'

'I understand what it feels like to let someone be who they are.'

'I know how to let someone be who they are.'

'I understand what it feels like when the world is in perfect harmony and balance.'

'I understand what it feels like to live my daily life without being overly critical of myself or others.'

Life Purpose

'I know the Creator's perspective on my life's purpose.'

'I know it is possible to know my life's purpose.'

Listening

'I understand the Creator's definition of listening.'

'I understand what it feels like to listen.'

'I know when to listen.'

'I know how to listen.'

'I know how to live my daily life listening.'

'I know the Creator's perspective on listening.'

'I know it is possible to be a good listener.'

'I understand what it feels like to be listened to by a man/woman/the Creator of All That Is.'

'I know how to be listened to by a man/woman/the Creator of All That Is.'

Love

'I understand the Creator's definition of love.'

'I understand what it feels like to love my fellow man/woman.'

'I know how to love my fellow man/woman.'

'I know the Creator's perspective on love.'

'I know it is possible to love my fellow man/woman.'

'I understand the definition of a mother's love through the Creator of All That Is.'

'I understand what it feels like to have a mother's love.'

'I know how to live my daily life with a mother's love.'

'I know the Creator's perspective on a mother's love.'

'I know it is possible to receive a mother's love.'

'I understand the Creator's definition of a father's love.'

'I understand what it feels like to have a father's love.'

'I know how to live my daily life with a father's love.'

'I know the Creator's perspective on a father's love.'

'I know it is possible to receive a father's love.'

Loving People for Who They Are

'I understand the Creator's definition of loving people for who they are.'

'I understand what it feels like to love people for who they are.'

'I know how to love people for who they are.'

'I know how to live my daily life with love.'

'I know the Creator's perspective on love.'

'I know it is possible to love people for who they are.'

Loyalty

'I understand the Creator's definition of loyalty.'

'I understand what it feels like to be loyal.'

'I know how to be loyal.'

'I know when to be loyal.'

'I know how to live my daily life in loyalty.'

'I know the Creator's perspective on loyalty.'

'I know it is possible to be loyal.'

Magic

'I understand the Creator's definition of magic.'

'I understand what it feels like to be magical.'

'I know how to be magical.'

'I know when to be magical.'

'I know how to live my daily life magically.'

'I know the Creator's perspective on magic.'

'I know it is possible to experience magic.'

Miracles

'I understand the Creator's definition of miracles.'

'I understand what a miracle feels like.'

'I know when a miracle happens.'

'I know how to manifest and witness miracles.'

'I know how to live my daily life with miracles.'

'I know the Creator's perspective on miracles.'

'I know it is possible to witness miracles.'

Money

'I understand what it feels like to have money.'

'I know how to have money.'

'I know how to live my daily life with money.'

'I know the Creator's perspective on money.'

'I know it is possible to have money.'

'I know that money is a form of exchange.'

Motivation

'I understand the Creator's definition of motivation.'

'I understand what it feels like to be motivated by the Creator of All That Is.'

'I know how to be motivated by the Creator of All That Is.'

'I know how to live my daily life with motivation.'

'I know the Creator's perspective on motivation.'

'I know it is possible to be motivated by the Creator of All That Is.'

Peace

'I understand the Creator's definition of peace.'

'I understand what it feels like to have peace.'

'I know how to have peace.'

'I know how to live my daily life in peace.'

'I know the Creator's perspective on peace.'

'I know it is possible to have peace.'

Perseverance

'I understand the Creator's definition of perseverance.'

'I understand what it feels like to persevere.'

'I know how to persevere.'

'I know it is possible to persevere.'

Play

> 'I understand the Creator's definition of how to play.'

> 'I understand what it feels like to play.'

> 'I know when to play.'

> 'I know how to play.'

> 'I know how to live my daily life in play.'

> 'I know the Creator's perspective on play.'

> 'I know it is possible to play.'

Pride

> 'I understand the Creator's definition of pride.'

> 'I understand what it feels like to be proud.'

> 'I know when to be proud.'

> 'I know how to be proud.'

> 'I know how to live my daily life with pride.'

> 'I know the Creator's perspective on pride.'

> 'I know it is possible to be proud.'

> 'I understand what it feels like to have pride in my work.'

Relaxation

> 'I understand the Creator's definition of relaxation.'

> 'I understand what it feels like to relax.'

> 'I know when to relax.'

> 'I know how to relax.'

> 'I know how to live my daily life relaxed.'

> 'I know the Creator's perspective on relaxation.'

> 'I know it is possible to relax.'

Resolving Programmes

'I understand what it feels like to find and resolve my own programmes.'

'I know how to find and resolve my own programmes.'

Respect

'I understand the Creator's definition of respect for myself and others.'

'I understand what it feels like to have respect for myself and others.'

'I know how to have respect for myself and others.'

'I know how to live my daily life with respect for all things.'

'I know the Creator's perspective on respect.'

'I know it is possible to have respect.'

'I understand what it feels like to be respected by my students.'

'I know how to be respected by my students.'

'I know it is possible to be respected by my students.'

Rest

'I understand the Creator's definition of rest.'

'I understand what it feels like to rest.'

'I know when to rest.'

'I know how to rest.'

'I know the Creator's perspective on rest.'

'I know it is possible to rest.'

Safety

'I understand the Creator's definition of safety.'

'I understand what it feels like to be safe.'

'I know when I am safe.'

'I know how to be safe.'

'I know how to live my daily life in safety.'

'I know the Creator's perspective on safety.'

'I know it is possible to be safe.'

Saying No

'I understand what it feels like to say no.'

'I know when to say no.'

'I know how to say no.'

'I know it is possible to say no.'

Security

'I understand the Creator's definition of security.'

'I understand what it feels like to be secure.'

'I know how to be secure.'

'I know how to live my daily life in security.'

'I know the Creator's perspective on security.'

'I know it is possible to be secure.'

Seeing Yourself Clearly

'I know how to see myself clearly according to the Creator's definition.'

'I know it is possible to see myself clearly according to the Creator's definition.'

Self-acceptance

'I understand the Creator's definition of self-acceptance.'

'I understand what it feels like to accept myself.'

'I know how to accept myself.'

'I know how to live my daily life accepting myself completely.'

'I know it is possible to accept myself completely.'

Serenity

'I understand the Creator's definition of serenity.'

'I understand what it feels like to be serene.'

'I know how to be serene.'

'I know how to live my daily life in serenity.'

'I know the Creator's perspective on serenity.'

'I know it is possible to be serene.'

Sons and Daughters

'I understand the Creator's definition of a son or daughter.'

'I understand what it feels like to be a son or daughter.'

'I know how to live my daily life as a son or daughter.'

'I know the Creator's perspective of a son or daughter.'

'I know it is possible to be a son or a daughter.'

Speaking

'I have something to say.'

'I have something worthwhile to say to others.'

'I know what I have to say is important.'

Speaking Your Truth

'I understand the Creator's definition of speaking my truth.'

'I understand what it feels like to speak my truth.'

'I know when to speak my truth.'

'I know how to speak my truth.'

'I know how to live my daily life speaking my truth.'

'I know it is possible to speak my truth.'

Stillness

'I understand the Creator's definition of stillness.'

'I understand what it feels like to be still.'

'I know when to be still.'

'I know how to be still.'

'I know how to live my daily life in stillness.'

'I know it is possible to be still.'

Success

'I understand the Creator's definition of success.'

'I understand what it feels like to succeed.'

'I know how to succeed.'

'I know how to live my daily life successfully.'

'I know the Creator's perspective on success.'

'I know it is possible to succeed.'

Tact

'I understand the Creator's definition of tact.'

'I understand what it feels like to be tactful.'

'I know how to be tactful.'

'I know how to live my daily life being tactful.'

'I know the Creator's perspective on tact.'

'I know it is possible to be tactful.'

Thankfulness

'I understand the Creator's definition of thankfulness.'

'I understand what it feels like to be thankful.'

'I know when to be thankful.'

'I know how to be thankful.'

'I know how to live my daily life thankfully.'

'I know the Creator's perspective on thankfulness.'

'I know it is possible to be thankful.'

Theta Work

'I understand what it feels like to do Theta work on myself.'

'I know when to do Theta work on myself.'

'I know how to do Theta work on myself.'

'I know how to live my daily life with the ability to do Theta work on myself.'

'I know it is possible to do Theta work on myself.'

Tranquillity

'I understand the Creator's definition of tranquillity.'

'I understand what it feels like to be tranquil.'

'I know how to be tranquil.'

'I know how to live my daily life in tranquillity.'

'I know the Creator's perspective on tranquillity.'

'I know it is possible to be tranquil.'

Trust

'I understand the Creator's definition of being trustworthy.'

'I understand what it feels like to be trustworthy.'

'I know how to be trustworthy.'

'I know it is possible to be trustworthy.'

'I understand the Creator's definition of trusting myself.'

'I understand what it feels like to trust myself 100 percent.'

'I know how to trust myself 100 percent.'

'I know it is possible to trust myself 100 percent.'

'I understand the Creator's definition of trust in the Creator.'

'I understand what it feels like to trust the Creator 100 percent.'

'I know how to trust the Creator 100 percent.'

'I know how to live my daily life with complete trust in the Creator.'

'I know it is possible to trust the Creator 100 percent.'

Truth

'I understand the Creator's definition of the highest truth.'

'I know how to live my daily life according to the highest truth.'

'I know the Creator's perspective on the highest truth.'

'I know it is possible to know the highest truth.'

'I know truth.'

'I know how to see truth.'

'I know how to live my daily life in truth.'

'I know it is possible to see truth.'

'I understand what it feels like to hear truth.'

'I know how to hear truth.'

'I know how to hear truth in my daily life.'

'I know it is possible to hear truth.'

'I understand what truth feels like.'

'I know it is possible to feel truth.'

'I understand what it feels like to smell truth.'

'I know what truth smells like.'

'I know how to smell truth.'

'I know it is possible to smell truth.'

Uniqueness

'I understand the Creator's definition of uniqueness.'

'I understand what it feels like to be unique.'

'I know how to be unique.'

'I know it is possible to be unique.'

Wisdom

> 'I understand the Creator's definition of wisdom.'
>
> 'I understand what it feels like to have wisdom.'
>
> 'I know when to have wisdom.'
>
> 'I know how to have wisdom.'
>
> 'I know how to live my daily life with wisdom.'
>
> 'I know the Creator's perspective on wisdom.'
>
> 'I know it is possible to have wisdom.'

More Feelings and Programmes!

In our day-to-day life we can use feeling work to explore knowledge and feelings we may not have. Using the following sentence structures, insert the feelings that you may need to instill in yourself or others:

> 'I know what it *feels like* to live without...'
>
> 'I know what it *feels like* and *I know how to live my day-to-day life* without...'
>
> 'I know what it *feels like* and *I know how to live my day-to-day life* without fear of...'
>
> 'I know what it *feels like* and *I know how to live my day-to-day life* without having to...'

Instill these feelings in yourself or help another person to accept them:

How to Live Without...

> 'I know what it feels like and I know how to live my day-to-day life without doubt.'
>
> 'I know what it feels like and I know how to live my day-to-day life without anger.'
>
> 'I know what it feels like and I know how to live my day-to-day life without fear.'
>
> 'I know what it feels like and I know how to live my day-to-day life without pain.'

'I know what it feels like and I know how to live my day-to-day life without sickness.'

'I know what it feels like and I know how to live my day-to-day life without resentment.'

'I know what it feels like and I know how to live my day-to-day life without holding grudges.'

'I know what it feels like and I know how to live my day-to-day life without regret.'

'I know what it feels like and I know how to live my day-to-day life without creating battle.'

'I know what it feels like and I know how to live my day-to-day life without being depressed.'

'I know what it feels like and I know how to live my day-to-day life without gloom and doom.'

'I know what it feels like and I know how to live my day-to-day life without disappointment.'

'I know what it feels like and I know how to live my day-to-day life without discouragement.'

'I know what it feels like and I know how to live my day-to-day life without drama.'

'I know what it feels like and I know how to live my day-to-day life without chaos.'

'I know what it feels like and I know how to live my day-to-day life without being pathetic.'

'I know what it feels like and I know how to live my day-to-day life without being pitiful.'

'I know what it feels like and I know how to live my day-to-day life without being hyper.'

'I know what it feels like and I know how to live my day-to-day life without being abused.'

'I know what it feels like and I know how to live my day-to-day life without being used.'

'I know what it feels like and I know how to live my day-to-day life without scarcity.'

'I know what it feels like and I know how to live my day-to-day life without envy.'

'I know what it feels like and I know how to live my day-to-day life without jealousy.'

'I know what it feels like and I know how to live my day-to-day life without coveting others.'

'I know what it feels like and I know how to live my day-to-day life without being impatient.'

'I know what it feels like and I know how to live my day-to-day life without being miserable.'

'I know what it feels like and I know how to live my day-to-day life without worry.'

'I know what it feels like and I know how to live my day-to-day life without despair.'

'I know what it feels like and I know how to live my day-to-day life without doubting my power.'

'I know what it feels like and I know how to live my day-to-day life without fear of seeing the truth.'

'I know what it feels like and I know how to live my day-to-day life without resentment.'

'I know what it feels like and I know how to live my day-to-day life without denial.'

'I know what it feels like and I know how to live my day-to-day life without being irritated.'

'I know what it feels like and I know how to live my day-to-day life without shame.'

'I know what it feels like and I know how to live my day-to-day life without confusion.'

'I know what it feels like and I know how to live my day-to-day life without stress.'

'I know what it feels like and I know how to live my day-to-day life without anxiety.'

'I know what it feels like and I know how to live my day-to-day life without being threatened.'

'I know what it feels like and I know how to live my day-to-day life without threatening others.'

'I know what it feels like and I know how to live my day-to-day life without allowing others to hurt me.'

'I know what it feels like and I know how to live my day-to-day life without allowing others to victimize me.'

'I know what it feels like and I know how to live my day-to-day life without being a victim.'

'I know what it feels like and I know how to live my day-to-day life without annoying others.'

'I know what it feels like and I know how to live my day-to-day life without irritating others.'

'I know what it feels like and I know how to live my day-to-day life without road rage.'

'I know what it feels like and I know how to live my day-to-day life without instability.'

'I know what it feels like and I know how to live my day-to-day life without being punished.'

'I know what it feels like and I know how to live my day-to-day life without being overwhelmed.'

'I know what it feels like and I know how to live my day-to-day life without being nervous about the next step forward.'

'I know what it feels like and I know how to live my day-to-day life without being nervous about the future.'

'I know what it feels like and I know how to live my day-to-day life without being angry with my family.'

'I know what it feels like and I know how to live my day-to-day life without being angry with myself.'

'I know what it feels like and I know how to live my day-to-day life without being angry with the Creator.'

'I know what it feels like and I know how to live my day-to-day life without my world falling apart.'

'I know what it feels like and I know how to live my day-to-day life without worrying about having enough time.'

'I know what it feels like and I know how to live my day-to-day life without taking on other people's "stuff".'

'I know what it feels like and I know how to live my day-to-day life without criticizing myself or others.'

'I know what it feels like and I know how to live my day-to-day life without making excuses for who I am.'

'I know what it feels like and I know how to live my day-to-day life without doubting my ability to see clearly in the body.'

'I know what it feels like and I know how to live my day-to-day life without buying into group conscious fear.'

'I know what it feels like and I know how to live my day-to-day life without punishing myself with food, cigarettes, drugs and alcohol.'

'I know what it feels like and I know how to live my day-to-day life without thinking it hurts to feel.'

'I know what it feels like and I know how to live my day-to-day life without being betrayed.'

'I know what it feels like and I know how to live my day-to-day life without being ignored.'

'I know what it feels like and I know how to live my day-to-day life without having to be miserable.'

'I know what it feels like and I know how to live my day-to-day life without having to forget.'

'I know what it feels like and I know how to live my day-to-day life without having to shut up.'

'I know what it feels like and I know how to live my day-to-day life without having to shut down.'

'I know what it feels like and I know how to live my day-to-day life without having to be the bad guy.'

'I know what it feels like and I know how to live my day-to-day life without having to allow the underdog to take advantage of me.'

'I know what it feels like and I know how to live my day-to-day life without having to be blamed for others' mistakes.'

'I know what it feels like and I know how to live my day-to-day life without having to cut myself off from All That Is.'

'I know what it feels like and I know how to live my day-to-day life without having to take on other people's suffering, but if I do, it changes to light and love instantly.'

How to Live Without Feeling...

'I know what it feels like and I know how to live my day-to-day life without feeling inferior.'

'I know what it feels like and I know how to live my day-to-day life without feeling lonely.'

'I know what it feels like and I know how to live my day-to-day life without feeling abandoned.'

'I know what it feels like and I know how to live my day-to-day life without feeling pessimistic.'

'I know what it feels like and I know how to live my day-to-day life without feeling neglected.'

'I know what it feels like and I know how to live my day-to-day life without feeling excluded.'

'I know what it feels like and I know how to live my day-to-day life without feeling left behind.'

'I know what it feels like and I know how to live my day-to-day life without feeling beaten up.'

'I know what it feels like and I know how to live my day-to-day life without feeling broken.'

'I know what it feels like and I know how to live my day-to-day life without feeling unimportant.'

'I know what it feels like and I know how to live my day-to-day life without feeling crazy.'

'I know what it feels like and I know how to live my day-to-day life without feeling stupid.'

'I know what it feels like and I know how to live my day-to-day life without feeling inferior.'

'I know what it feels like and I know how to live my day-to-day life without feeling belittled.'

'I know what it feels like and I know how to live my day-to-day life without feeling disregarded.'

'I know what it feels like and I know how to live my day-to-day life without feeling minimized.'

'I know what it feels like and I know how to live my day-to-day life without feeling like a burden.'

'I know what it feels like and I know how to live my day-to-day life without feeling burdened.'

'I know what it feels like and I know how to live my day-to-day life without feeling like a bother.'

'I know what it feels like and I know how to live my day-to-day life without feeling shunned.'

'I know what it feels like and I know how to live my day-to-day life without feeling that I'm in the wrong family.'

'I know what it feels like and I know how to live my day-to-day life without feeling that I'm on the wrong planet.'

'I know what it feels like and I know how to live my day-to-day life without feeling that I'm in the wrong body.'

'I know what it feels like and I know how to live my day-to-day life without feeling responsible for my parents.'

'I know what it feels like and I know how to live my day-to-day life without feeling out of control.'

'I know what it feels like and I know how to live my day-to-day life without feeling like I am the parent of my parents.'

'I know what it feels like and I know how to live my day-to-day life without feeling threatened.'

How to Live Without the Fear Of…

'I know what it feels like and I know how to live my day-to-day life without the fear of being disconnected from the Creator.'

'I know what it feels like and I know how to live my day-to-day life without the fear of falling back asleep and forgetting the truth.'

'I know what it feels like and I know how to live my day-to-day life without the fear of failing my mission in this life.'

'I know what it feels like and I know how to live my day-to-day life without the fear of intimacy.'

'I know what it feels like and I know how to live my day-to-day life without the fear of being vulnerable with others.'

'I know what it feels like and I know how to live my day-to-day life without the fear of being awesome.'

'I know what it feels like and I know how to live my day-to-day life without the fear of God.'

6

ADVANCED BELIEF, FEELING AND DIGGING WORK

Our brain works like a biological super-computer, assessing information and responding to it. *How* we respond depends on the information that we receive and how we interpret it – whether it becomes a belief system. When a belief has been accepted as real by the body, mind or soul, it becomes a programme.

Programmes can be to our benefit or detriment, depending on what they are and how we are reacting to them. In their negative form, they can have adverse effects on our heart, mind, body and soul.

BELIEF WORK

Belief work empowers people with the ability to remove these negative programmes and belief systems and replace them with positive ones from the Creator of All That Is. It is a means of changing behaviour. The behaviour may be physical, mental or spiritual in nature.

This also enables healing to happen. I was shown that for healing to take place, the person receiving it must want to be restored to health and the person giving it must believe it is possible, otherwise it will be impossible for them to witness it. In both cases, belief work will help.

One of the best ways to change beliefs is through a return to the purity of a child. When we are children, our brainwave pattern is open to receiving and accepting new information. This is why the Theta state is so important, as it returns the subconscious to that frequency of growth and change and opens the mind to positive change.

When we are children, we are receptive to changing belief systems, but as adults we do not easily access the subconscious mind without hours of therapy or hypnosis. Belief work is a means to do just that: access the subconscious mind. However, it also takes us a step further: it gives us the ability to change beliefs that go beyond the subconscious into the spiritual and genetic areas, which are largely ignored in alternative therapy.

THE FOUR BELIEF LEVELS

I teach in ThetaHealing that we are creating our own life adventure and are allowed to change our beliefs. All we have to do is to go to the right place to change them.

I have already explained in the *ThetaHealing* book that there are four 'belief levels', but it is worth briefly recapping the information here.

The four belief levels within the All That Is of a person comprise their body, emotions, mind and even the expansiveness of their soul energy. These belief systems extend into the past, present and future, even to the electromagnetic energy that tells the DNA what to do. They are the basis of the belief work.

The Core Belief Level

Core beliefs are what we are taught and accept from childhood in this life. They are beliefs that have become a part of us. They are held as energy in the frontal lobe of the brain.

The Genetic Level

At this level, programmes are carried over from ancestors or added to our genes in this life. These energies are stored in the morphogenetic field around the physical DNA. This 'field' of knowledge is what tells the mechanics of the DNA what to do. This belief level can be accessed through the master cell in the pineal gland of the brain.

The History Level

This level concerns memories from past lives or deep genetic memory or collective consciousness experiences that we carry into the present. These memories are held in our auric field.

The Soul Level

This level is all that we are. Here the programmes are pulled off our complete being, beginning at the heart chakra and moving outward.

◇◇◇◇◇

A belief programme can exist on one or more of the levels or simultaneously on all four. If it is removed from one level and not the others, it will simply replace itself on that level. This is why it is necessary to pull it from all the levels. This also creates a change on all the planes of existence.

When I want a programme to be pulled, I go up above my space and ask the Creator to pull it on all four levels. Then I witness it being released and a new programme coming in from the purity of the divine.

In *ThetaHealing* I taught you how to release belief programmes from each individual level and then from all the levels simultaneously. Once the advanced practitioner becomes familiar with recognizing what a belief programme is and how many levels it resides on, the process becomes much faster. The human brain works much more quickly than we realize. When you become familiar with belief work, programmes will be sent to the Creator and replaced at the speed of thought.

BELIEF WORK PRINCIPLES

Here's a short list to remind you of the principles of belief work:

Verbal Permission

Always remember that the person receiving the belief work must give full verbal permission to the practitioner to *remove and replace programmes* and full verbal permission to the practitioner for *each and every programme*. We have the free agency to keep any belief programmes we choose. Another person cannot change programmes without our verbal permission. It will not work.

Preserving Programmes and Beliefs

Be very careful what programmes that you release. Some programmes are for our benefit.

For example, when I was a little girl I remember coming to the realization, 'These people can't love me. I'm going to have to love them. I'm going to have to teach them how to love me.'

Understanding this programme has shown me why I am the person that I am and also why I've done what I've done in my life. Upon reflection, I realized it wasn't such a bad programme. I thought to myself, 'I think that I will keep part of this programme, the part of "I know how to love others".'

Some of your beliefs have got you where you are today. Be gentle with yourself.

'Programme Did Not Hold'

I have heard that some practitioners have changed a programme over and over again and the new programme has not 'held' – the person hasn't retained it. This will be because they haven't known what it *feels like*.

For instance, if I go in to a person's space and the Creator gives them the programme 'I know I am loved', it's not going to hold to the next day if they don't know what it *feels like to be loved*. This is where the feeling work comes in. So, if I go up and say, 'Creator of All That Is, show this person what love feels like,' then all the programmes that I give them will hold. When I do this, I envisage the feeling pouring down like a waterfall on all the levels until it's in every cell of their body. Then the body knows what it feels like to be loved.

Programmes can definitely be changed in this way. However, they can be re-created by the things we say, think and do (or choose not to do). *Positive action* is needed to change our lives.

Clearing your Mind

First work on the beliefs that clear your mind. That way you can find the bottom belief, the one that you need to change.

If you are ill, ask the Creator, 'Which beliefs do I need to work on to heal this sickness?' You may be told that you need to release a particular belief system, but you need to clear your mind as well.

Communicating with the Subconscious Mind

Remember that the subconscious mind doesn't understand words like 'don't', 'isn't', 'can't' and 'not'. You should tell the client to omit these words in their statements when in the belief work process. For example, they should not use a statement such as 'I don't love myself' or 'I can't love myself'.

To properly test for a programme, the statement should be 'I love myself' and the client will energy test positive or negative.

Dual Beliefs

If you find a person who has a dual belief system – for example, a person who believes they are rich but at the same time believes they are poor – leave the positive programme in place and pull the negative programme, replacing it with the correct positive one from the Creator.

Pulling Negative Programmes

You can never command all negative programmes to leave the body because the subconscious mind does not know which programmes are negative or positive.

Death Wishes

Some important programmes to watch for in belief work sessions are death wishes. The Creator told me that many people have death wishes, but not all death wishes should be randomly pulled and replaced. For instance, an old Viking belief is that you should have a good death. If you pull this kind of genetic programme the person may begin to feel that they don't want to live anymore, because to them, death is a part of living.

On a genetic level, some nationalities, such as the Japanese and Native Americans, believe in an honourable death. This is a good example of a negative belief system serving a person.

Words Have Power

Listen to what you say! The spoken word is incredibly powerful in a belief work session. Remember that if you find that a woman hates men, you should not programme her with 'I release all men' or she may leave her spouse and never be with another male. Pay careful attention to what you are suggesting.

Working Alone or with a Practitioner

Some of the programmes we carry have emotional attachments to them. So when you are removing programmes from yourself, it may be rewarding to allow someone to assist you in the process. Working with an experienced ThetaHealing practitioner is helpful, since the practitioner can guide you in the proper replacement of programmes while remaining emotionally detached. However, some people are comfortable working on themselves. It all depends on the individual.

Ask the Creator

When teaching belief work I am often asked, 'What do you replace the negative programme with?' My answer is always the same: 'Ask the Creator.' Replacement beliefs should always be divinely inspired.

Remember, the Creator will help you with *anything* if you keep your *ego* out of the equation.

ENERGY TESTING

For the ThetaHealing beginner, energy testing – testing a person's subconscious to find if they have certain belief programmes – is a crucial tool. Energy testing allows both the practitioner and the client to see, through a reaction to stimuli, that a belief programme exists and, once the belief work is complete, that it has been changed and a new one is in place. (For step-by-step instructions in energy testing, refer to *ThetaHealing* or applied kinaesiology books.)

When you become experienced in one-on-one belief work sessions, you won't need energy testing to know that a belief has cleared. You may still energy-test, however, so that the client can see what their beliefs are and that they've changed. Energy testing is also used as a reminder not to become egotistical and forget to look for the answer.

BELIEF SYSTEMS CONNECTED TO EMOTIONS

The natural emotions of the human condition are different from programmes. Remember that emotions are natural. Most of the time, they are for our benefit. Our true emotions – *anger*, *love*, *sorrow*, *happiness* and *fear* – can actually save our lives. All of them are at one time or another necessary for our wellbeing. Therefore, we do not attempt to pull *all that an emotion is* from a person.

However, when emotions such as anger and sorrow are allowed to go unchecked and get out of control, they have a negative impact on our body. They can also endlessly loop through the mind, begging to be set free. It is permissible to pull and replace these emotions, since they have become belief systems.

Emotions can also be changed or altered by the toxins and chemical reactions of the body. Altering the DNA of the body can change these chemical reactions.

REJECTION, RESENTMENT, REGRET

I believe that emotions and thought forms can create 'emotional molecules' that become a physical essence in the body. These molecules can exert a toll in all kinds of ways. One of them is the hampering of our intuitive abilities. The reason we don't have all of our psychic abilities available to us is because we are harbouring too many resentments and grudges, either ones that we have created or ones that have been handed down to us. It takes time, space and energy to maintain resentments, and certain areas in the brain are being occupied by this energy.

I believe that resentment, regret and rejection have considerable influence over us and have a direct connection to the beliefs that block the body from healing. Analyzing a person for beliefs associated with resentment, regret and rejection can change the outcome of their session. It is important to follow through on this.

Never underestimate the power of the human mind. The unconscious mind knows that a person can use resentment to prevent something worse from happening. For instance, when a person resents their father, they may be saving themselves from abandonment or abuse. So the mind is choosing resentment as the lesser of two evils. The problem lies in the fact that the mind will replay that programme and create more resentment in a constant effort to protect itself. Pulling and replacing the programme of 'I resent my father' will relieve the resentment somewhat. But once the receptors of the brain have been taught to expect constant resentment, the person will find someone else to resent and this will keep the belief intact.

To take another example, in the past I needed someone to tell me that I couldn't do something. I would always say to these people, 'I *can* do it, watch me!' It was almost as if I needed someone to say something was *impossible* just so that I could prove to them that I could do it. It seemed that I would bring people into my life to tell me I couldn't do something. But these people served a purpose: I'd use their reaction to give me the motivation to achieve. As soon as I cleared the beliefs associated with the need to be told I couldn't do something, I realized that the need for these *people* in my life had changed. Changing my beliefs changed my relationships with the people around me.

People come into our life to show us beliefs, programmes and feelings that need to be released and/or instilled. So, if you are bringing someone into your life who is abusive in some way, look for the reason for it. You may be using an abusive situation as an excuse to not go forward. I've had people tell me over and over again that it is their husbands or their wives who keep them from going forward. This is just using another person as an excuse. Releasing the programme of 'I need someone to challenge me' will change the relationship. The person will no longer be projecting their programmes onto their spouse and so these qualities will not be brought out in the spouse.

Relationships are based on emotions and programmes that are projected onto the other person. Some relationships bring out good emotions; others bring out harsh and cruel emotions. But whatever the reason for the relationship, it will be serving the person in some way.

Some people go through their lives with the programme of 'Everyone I love hurts me'. If you have this programme, you may push people away and they may respond in the very way that you do not want them to respond.

One programme that I found that I had was that I didn't know how to receive love from a man. Once I found that I had this programme, I realized that in all the relationships that I had been in, I had been loved but had not known how to receive it. I realized that no matter how many people try to love you, if you don't know how to permit yourself to *receive* it, you can't *accept* it.

GRUDGES

I used being told I couldn't do something to motivate myself into action, but a lot of people use grudges. Some people carry them from their ancestors and don't even know that they have them, but others bear conscious grudges towards places, the government, their partner, themselves and what they haven't accomplished.

If you have a grudge against a partner, you should ask yourself how it is serving you.

When a grudge is pulled and released, the space will be filled by God's light and result in enhanced psychic abilities.

Test for the following beliefs and download the following feelings if needed:

Grudges: Beliefs

'I like my grudges.'

'My grudges protect me.'

'Without grudges, people will take advantage of me.'

Grudges: Feelings Downloads

'I know what it feels like to live without grudges.'

'I know how to live without grudges.'

'I know how to live and be safe without grudges.'

WORRY

Worry is very hard on your system. It will throw your serotonin levels off-balance and can cause stomach problems. You can develop irritable bowel syndrome if you are worried all the time.

Most people don't know how to live without worry. In fact, some people begin to feel that if they aren't worried about something they aren't living! But if you realized how much time you spent worrying, you would understand how much energy you are wasting on it. Teach yourself to know how to live without worry – this energy should be spent in constructive endeavours.

If you begin to get nervous when I suggest you live without worry, it is likely to be because you think you aren't going to 'worry' about things like paying your bills. These things have to do with *responsibility*. I'm not saying you shouldn't be responsible. You can be responsible and not have excess worry all the time.

Some people need stress and drama to make life more exciting. It is easy to become addicted to stress and the creation of drama. But when you instill the feeling of 'I know how to live without stress and drama', it will release you from the addiction to these energies.

DIGGING WORK

One of the ways in which you can be more effective in a one-on-one session is to use the digging technique. As you know, this locates the bottom belief that is holding up many other beliefs.

One of the most prevalent questions that I am asked by my students is: 'How do you know *when* to use the digging work?' My answer is simpler than you might think. You see, you really don't have to know when, or how, to do the digging work. The subconscious mind of the client will do all the work for you. All you have to remember is to ask 'Who?', 'What?', 'Where?', 'Why?' and 'How?' The client's mind will do the digging for you, accessing information like a computer, and will give you an answer to every question. If the client seems to get stuck, it will only be temporary. Change the question you are asking. If there is no still answer, ask them, 'If you *did* know an answer, what would it be?' With a little practice, you will learn how to use your intuition to find the answer.

The key is to listen to what the person is saying. Issues that are repeated or cause great emotion are usually related to the bottom belief. Listen to your client very closely and they will give you big clues to the answers to their dilemmas.

Also, at any time in the belief work process, the Creator may come to you and give you the bottom belief that you are looking for, so be open to divine intervention.

Here is a brief recap of the process:

1. Ask the person, 'If there is anything you would change in your life, what would it be?' Then ask them questions about the issue they come up with until you have reached the deepest core issue. You will know that you are close to the key belief when they begin to become verbally defensive, wriggle or cry in a subconscious attempt to hold on to the programme. Pull, cancel, resolve and replace the issue as necessary on whatever belief levels you have found it, using the key questions 'Who?', 'What?', 'Where?', 'Why?' and 'How?'

2. Avoid putting your own programmes or feelings into the investigation process.

3. Be sure you are firmly connected to the perspective of the Creator of the Seventh Plane when you are in the person's space. In some instances, they will loop, hide or take you in circles with the question/answer scenario. Be patient and persistent. It may be necessary to ask the Creator what the deeper programme is.

You can tell when you are nearing the bottom belief when the person's energy tests positive with their eyes open and their eyes closed.

As you begin to reach the bottom belief, it is easy to interpret some of the beliefs directly above it as being the bottom belief, and this can be confusing. It is important to watch the client's body language and listen closely to what they are saying. As you get closer to the bottom belief, they will become increasingly uncomfortable, because you are triggering, releasing and resolving *trauma*.

As well as looking for the bottom belief, you are also searching for the *positive benefit* that the person may be getting from having that bottom belief.

You should also find out what happened in their life to give rise to the bottom belief.

When you find and release the bottom belief, your client should feel renewed. They should be refreshed and empowered. If they get up from the session with aches and pains or don't feel better, then you haven't finished the belief work. Understand that a person may need more than one belief work session in order to find the bottom issues.

The digging process is one of the most important things in ThetaHealing. Some students, for example, when they start using the belief and feeling work, will start downloading all the beliefs and feelings possible, thinking this is going to help them. In a certain sense they are right, but not to the extent they expect. What this does is *add to* the feelings and beliefs that are already there. What it does *not* do is find the bottom beliefs – the ones that really need to be removed and replaced – and all the particular feelings that are truly needed.

Many practitioners and teachers of ThetaHealing have made lists and lists of feelings that they wish to have instillled in themselves and in others. Some of them have sat down and worked on thousands of beliefs, but neglected to use the digging work. However, releasing beliefs at random without finding the bottom belief will only cause confusion.

The same is true with diseases. Some people come to me and tell me they have pulled every belief that they can possibly clear that is associated with their disease. They say that it works for everyone else, but not for them. The truth most likely is that they have not cleared the bottom beliefs associated with the sickness and do not want to take the time to look for them. What they have done is sit down with a list of beliefs compiled by someone else that may not pertain to them. Every one of us is special; our diseases and beliefs are special to us. *Although there might be similarities in the beliefs associated with a particular illness, each person is different, and we should never assume that the bottom beliefs is the same for everyone.* This is why I take a broad view about the belief systems associated with disease and believe it is best to listen to the client.

The beliefs associated with illness can be a simple challenge to overcome, however. Once the disease is gone, the real challenge is to help the person develop the ability to communicate with the Creator.

In essence, *ThetaHealing is all about teaching another person how to use the belief work to heal themselves.* It is also about changing your own beliefs to make your connection with the Creator the clearest it can be. It is about learning that all diseases and all problems in life can be changed. With simple decisions and a little belief work, your life and the lives of your clients can be changed forever.

REACTION TO BELIEFS

Remember that once you are in the process of seeking a key belief, it must be found before the end of the session or the person may experience a healing crisis. Do not leave them before their belief work is complete, and closely observe them for signs of discomfort. If they feel or act unsettled, or feel any pain or sorrow, then their issues have not been taken care of and the belief work should continue.

If a client experiences inexplicable physical pain in a session it is likely that you are reaching deep subconscious programmes. This means that you are triggering different belief systems that their subconscious is fighting to hold on to. Continue releasing beliefs until the pain has gone. With the person's permission, ask them to download what it *feels like* to be safe. Continue with the session until they are comfortable and have a peaceful demeanour.

GENETIC PROGRAMMES AND CORE BELIEFS

Another way of working on beliefs is to ask a person about the core beliefs that they may have accepted from their father and mother or that have passed down through the genes. To do this, energy test the client for programmes that they have inherited from their parents. For instance, their father might have been bossy and controlling. Energy test for the genetic programme of 'I am bossy and controlling like my father'.

Inheriting genetic beliefs from your parents does not mean that you will automatically enact them in your life. They may lie dormant and not manifest until they are triggered by the right set of circumstances. But whatever the case, these programmes can be cleared by exploring the beliefs of your parents and ancestors, and you will find that once they are gone you will be much more able to be successful in life.

Some of these genetic programmes could be 'The harder I work, the better things are' or 'I am poor and proud of it'. If you come from a family background without money, energy test yourself for:

'I am poor and proud of it.'

'I work hard for whatever I get.'

'It's wrong to be rich.'

Look at the things that your father and mother used to say and enact in their lives and test yourself for the related programmes, for example:

'I inherited my father's aggression.'

'I inherited my father's over-controlling behaviour.'

'I inherited my father's need for control.'

'I inherited my father's need to make everyone miserable.'

You should aim to be clear of these things before they enact themselves in your life!

OATHS AND COMMITMENTS

One of the contributions that my ThetaHealing instructors have given our modality is the exploration of the parameters of belief work. Some of my students have pushed the limits and experimented with aspects of the belief work by commanding that *all* oaths and commitments be removed from their past, present and future lives. This, in retrospect, is not necessarily a good thing, because some commitments and oaths might be for a person's benefit, or a person might want to keep them. Removing all of them is similar to removing large portions of the personality and leaving a void instead. It is therefore important to be specific about which oaths or commitments are removed. In removing commitments, I always command them to be *completed* and *finished* instead of arbitrarily removing those I choose to change.

In the past, a medical doctor that we were associated with suggested that we use a form of the Hippocratic oath for our teachers in order to instill some kind of responsibility and conscientiousness on their part towards the modality and their practice to others. Because ThetaHealing empowers people to remove oaths and commitments that are not serving them, asking people to declare an oath of allegiance to the modality and to themselves met with opposition on the part of some teachers, who felt that such an act would limit them in some way. The suggested oath was therefore removed from the ThetaHealing criteria due to the confusion and insecurity.

The point is, I have never said that oaths or commitments are bad *in themselves, only that some of them may not be serving us.* Some are good, for instance the vow of matrimony. So you should not pull all oaths and vows from this life, or from past lives either, since some of these programmes make up who and what you are. Always ask the Creator what should be pulled.

PROGRAMMES FROM GENETIC BELIEFS,
PAST LIVES AND GROUP CONSCIOUSNESS

Genetic beliefs can also show up in prejudice, for example: 'I am prejudiced against and offended by religions, ethnic groups, people who are different, people who are intellectual and people who are intellectually challenged.' The ThetaHealing World Relations course teaches you to energy-test yourself for these programmes.

Belief work can also be done by digging on subjects that relate to different times and places. If in the digging process you find that the source of the issue takes you to different times and places, ask yourself (or your client) what you learned from these experiences. If one of these issues has to do with abuse, for example, 'It's OK to let someone pick on me because I am strong', energy test to see if it comes from a past life.

As well as past lives, programmes can come from group consciousness. These are beliefs that have been accepted as valid by a large segment of the population and have therefore pervaded the collective consciousness of humanity. An example of a group consciousness belief would be 'Diabetes is incurable'.

POSITIVE BELIEFS CREATING A NEGATIVE OUTCOME

The important thing with digging work is to find how the issue is serving the person. It is the same thing with illness. If you can't find a reason why a person's illness is serving them, it is not likely that that illness will clear.

Illness is usually held in place by a *positive* belief. Many women with breast cancer, for example, believe on an unconscious level that the disease will bring their family closer together. They may believe on a subconscious level that it will help their relationships with their husband and children, bringing them all together in love and security. This is why they have to keep the illness.

There are also instances where a client's injuries, dysfunctional behaviour and negative programmes are serving them, albeit in an irrational fashion.

Energy test the client to discover whether they have hidden programmes that serve their disease or challenge by having them say, 'My [disease or challenge] is serving me.'

Then determine how it is happening by searching for the deepest programme and connecting to the Creator to pull and replace it.

NEGATIVE FEELINGS CREATING NEGATIVE RESULTS

The Danger of Downloading Negative Feelings

I am constantly reminded that belief work is incredibly powerful. An example of this came from some of my more senior teachers who were creating belief books compiled from their sessions and classes over the years. Since they were practical and careful ThetaHealers, they were intuitive enough to want it edited for content, and gave it to me. When I looked at the downloads and beliefs, I saw discrepancies. These pertained to downloads in the form of negative feelings to create a positive result. For instance, one person was suggesting downloading what depression felt like.

I realized that we might think that the Creator would give us the perspective of depression to benefit us and teach us how *not* to be depressed, but we are given exactly what we ask for, so if we ask to know the feeling of depression, then that is exactly what we will get: *the absolute pure essence of depression*. It follows that if the subconscious mind asks for a negative feeling, that is exactly what it is going to accept and create. This is the essence of co-creation between a person and the All That Is.

This is why we should avoid downloading negative feelings in an effort to create a positive result and should use positive feelings instead. In this case, for instance, a much better feeling download would be 'I know how to live without being depressed' or 'I know what it feels like to live without depression'.

Some instructors argue that they can download a negative feeling or thought and then later counter it with a positive programme. But it may take a week, a month or even a year for the negative feeling to melt away. And why would you want to know the Creator's definition of depression, of poverty or of sickness if this is exactly what you will get?

... and Some Positive Downloads

On the other side of the coin, there are some positive downloads that may also cause stress. An example of this would be 'I know how to deal with conflict'. This download will be likely to bring conflict, since that is exactly what you are asking for.

Remember the power of a feeling, thought or spoken word to manifest change. This change is generally straightforward and direct in nature. We get just what we ask for in the purest form.

Another download that would bring stress would be to ask to be completely independent and at the same time ask for a soulmate to share your life. This is an example of two programmes conflicting.

Think before you use the belief and feeling work.

7

DIGGING WORK SESSIONS

A few examples of digging work have already been given in *ThetaHealing*, but here are some that illustrate how deeply you need to work to clear an issue. Some practitioners fall short of finding the bottom belief and the feeling that needs to be instilled. It is better to keep digging…

Sitting across from the client, the first thing that you need to do is to ask them what they want to work on. Most people know exactly what it is before they ever sit down with you. Most of the topics that will come up will pertain to abundance, health or love.

One way to achieve amazing results is to start with what the client wants the outcome to be. A few examples of this follow, all taken from ThetaHealing certification classes with my students.

DIGGING WORK EXAMPLE 1: CANCER

Vianna to class: 'The first thing that you say to your client is: "What would you like to work on?"'

Client: 'I want to get better. I'm tired of being sick. I want the cancer gone.'

Vianna: 'Why are you sick?'

Client: 'I don't know why. I just want to be well.'

Vianna: *'But if you did know* why you were sick, *why* would it be?'

Client, becoming agitated: 'I don't know!'

At this point the practitioner should realize that this direction may be a dead end and begin a different course of questioning.

Vianna: '*What* is the best thing that has happened to you since you became sick?'

Client: 'There is nothing good. I've suffered and suffered.'

Vianna: '*But if there were something good* that came from you being sick, *what* would it be?'

Client: 'Well, my family gets along better now. My mother calls me and I'm able to talk to my father. I hadn't spoken to him in 15 years before this. I suppose you could say that our relationships have improved. This is the best thing that's happened since I've been sick.'

Vianna: 'Would your relationship with your parents continue to improve if you became healthy again?'

Client: 'No, no, I'm sure that everything would go back to what it was before.'

Vianna: 'So, really, it benefits you to be sick.'

Client: 'No ... well, I guess so, at least as far as my relationship with my parents is concerned.'

Vianna: 'Would you like to know that you can still have a relationship with your family without being sick?'

Client: 'Yes, I would!'

Here I download into the client the programme 'What it feels like to have a relationship with my family without being sick'. This does not indicate that the belief work session is finished, however. Since disease is usually created by more than one belief programme, I continue to question the client:

Vianna: 'What is the worst thing that would happen if you were better?'

Client: 'I would have to go back to work and I don't have a job. My finances are a mess and I can't take care of myself. Right now I'm getting benefits.'

Vianna: 'Would you like to know that there are other ways of solving this problem and that there are possibilities that you're not looking at?'

Client: 'Yes, I would!'

Since the client does not know how to create new opportunities, the feeling work is once again used. With the client's verbal permission, I download into him what it feels like to have possibilities, to recognize possibilities and to know that he can go back to work again. These are some of the bottom beliefs, but more digging might be necessary.

In many instances, as already mentioned, disease and other challenges are held by a positive belief instead of a negative belief. Here is an example of a positive belief bringing challenges:

DIGGING WORK EXAMPLE 2: LOOKING FOR LOVE

Vianna: 'What is it you would like to work on today?'

Client: 'I want to work on the fact that I can never find anyone to share my life with. I'm always alone. I can never find anyone to be with.'

Vianna: 'Why are you always alone?'

Client: 'I don't know. I can't figure it out. I'm a good person, I'm nice and I have no idea why I'm alone.'

Vianna: '*But if you did know* why you were alone, *what* would the answer be?'

At this point the client cannot come up with an answer and shrugs her shoulders. Now is the time to shift gears and change the course of the session.

Vianna: 'What is the best thing that happens when you are alone?'

Client: 'What do you mean, the *best thing* that happens when I'm alone?!'

Vianna: 'What I mean is, how does being alone benefit you?'

Client: 'Well, I know what I like to do with my time, and when you're in a relationship you always have to do what your partner wants to do. You don't ever get your own say-so. The other person seems to run your life.'

Vianna: 'Has this been your experience in past relationships?'

Client: 'Yes, this has been my experience. You can never be who you really are when you're in a relationship. You have to change to please the other person. You can't be yourself.'

Vianna: 'So, really, it's safer for you to be alone so that you can be yourself. Is this true?'

I energy-test the client for the programme of 'It's safe for me to be alone; at least then I can be myself'. She tests 'Yes' and begins to cry.

Client: 'I'm afraid to be with anyone. I'm afraid that they'll try to change me.'

Vianna: 'Would you like to know that there's someone out there who can accept you for who you really are and that you know how to be yourself with them so that you don't have to pretend to be something you're not?'

Client: 'Yes, I would!'

I connect to the Creator and, with permission, witness as these feelings are downloaded into her:

'I know how to be myself.'

'I know how to be considerate of the feelings of another person.'

'I understand how to share my feelings.'

'I understand how to share my life.'

'I understand what it feels like to share intimacy.'

'I know what it feels like to be intimate and kind.'

'I know how to allow someone into my life.'

Afterwards, the client begins to cry. Knowing that this is an old childhood programme, I can now continue in two ways. The first way is to ask the client:

Vianna: 'When was the first time you felt this way about relationships?'

Client: 'When my father left me.'

Vianna: 'Why did your father leave you?'

Client: 'I don't know. Everyone who loves me leaves me.'

This is also a bottom belief. I must now teach the client that it is possible to love another person without being abandoned. Depending upon the situation, I may also teach what it is like to be able to forgive and to understand the bigger picture. These are all possible downloads to use in this situation.

Vianna: 'What was positive about your father leaving you?'

Client: 'I learned to never trust a man and to do things myself.'

At this point the client is downloaded with 'I know how to share my life with someone' and 'It is possible to trust a man'. She feels uplifted and happy and the session is finished.

DIGGING WORK EXAMPLE 3:
LOVE, ABUNDANCE AND MOTHER ISSUES

Before you start digging work you really have to know what kind of outcome the person needs from the belief work session. The way that I do it is to have them sit very quietly and go up and connect to the Creator of All That Is and imagine exactly what they want in their life. I have them imagine exactly what they want in all aspects of their life as if they were truly living their dreams. I have them visualize that they're actually present in this abundance and that they have all their heart's desires. In some of these sessions the client desires material things such as cars, beautiful homes and lots of money. In this case, we are in a belief work session with a man who is about 35 years old.

Vianna: 'If you could have everything you ever wanted, what would it be?'

Man: 'I want three houses, one on the beach, lots of cars and plenty of money.'

Vianna: 'What would be the worst thing that could happen if you had all these things?'

This is a negative question to find the direction to the bottom belief. The reaction that you will get in a large majority of people will be one of fear and panic. After the fear and panic, the person will become crestfallen. This man was no different.

Man: 'If all this were really mine, I would be alone. There would be no one to share it with. It would be ridiculous to have all this and have no one to share it with, but that's the way it would be. I would be alone.'

Vianna: 'Why would you be alone?'

Man: 'I don't know how to get along with women.'

Vianna: 'Why can't you get along with women?'

Man: 'They don't understand me and I certainly don't understand them. It's better to give up before I even try.'

Vianna: 'Why do you say that?'

Man: 'Because once they know me, they tear me apart and put me down.'

Vianna: 'When did this start?'

Man: 'It started when I was little. My mother did it to me all the time.'

At this point I need to be careful to avoid becoming mired in programmes that pertain specifically to the man's mother – for example, 'My mother tortures me' – as these are not likely to be the bottom belief.

Vianna: 'What did your mother do to you?'

Man: 'I would do something that I thought was wonderful and I would run up to show her what I'd done. She would act as if it was nothing and shrug me off. I knew from that point on that I would never please a woman. So why should I try?'

Vianna: 'What did you learn from this?'

Man: 'I learned that it's ridiculous to even try.'

Vianna: 'Is this what your mother taught you?'

Man: 'My mother taught me not to trust anyone.'

Vianna: 'So if you don't trust anyone, what does that do for you?'

Man: 'Well, it keeps me from getting hurt. As long as I don't trust someone, they don't hurt me. And that's what I learned from my mother. I guess I should thank her for that.'

Now we have found the bottom belief: 'If I don't trust someone, they can't hurt me.' The first thing to do is to teach the person what it feels like to know whom to trust, when to trust, that it's possible to trust and how to trust without being hurt. The replacement feeling programme might be 'I know how to let someone love me and how to love them in return without being betrayed or betraying another'.

It is very important for the practitioner to stick with the belief work session until they reach the final outcome. It is very easy to become sidetracked before reaching the bottom belief.

Belief work doesn't have to take hours, though. In this case we found the bottom belief quickly. It was actually serving this man in some way. If he didn't let anyone into his life, he didn't have to trust. If he didn't have to trust, he didn't get hurt. He believed on a deep unconscious level that if he manifested everything that he wanted, he would ultimately end up alone. Ultimately, that was the reason why he didn't feel comfortable manifesting everything that his conscious mind wanted. This was what was stopping him. Once this issue had been cleared and he had been taught how to share his life with a partner, his manifesting abilities increased exponentially.

I find that in most instances people cannot manifest what they want because they don't *know* what they want. And nine times out of ten, sick people can't get better because they have never made plans to be healthy. What happens with most people is that the brain has only one goal in mind and that is to get through the day! This is particularly true when someone is very sick.

> *Stimulating people to think ahead to a point in their lives when they are healthy will bring up the issues that keep them from getting well.*

Once these issues have been brought to light, the practitioner has something to work on. Let's use an example of a person who wants to have abundance in their life:

DIGGING WORK EXAMPLE 4:
ABUNDANCE AND ISSUES WITH MOTHER

Vianna: 'If you could have everything you ever wanted, what would it be?'

Client: 'My dream is to own three houses, one in California, the others in New York and Paris. Each of the houses is lavishly furnished and in a beautiful location. I want to be able to travel all over the world to exotic locations, and I want to be strong and healthy.'

Vianna: 'How do you feel now that you have all this abundance? How do you feel now that all this is going to come into your life?'

Suddenly the client looks very nervous.

Client: 'I don't like the feeling of having all this.'

Vianna: 'Why don't you like the feeling of having all this?'

Client: 'Because everyone will be angry with me.'

Vianna: 'Why will everyone be angry with you?'

Client: 'Because I'll have more than everyone else that is in my life.'

Vianna: 'What feelings do you have because of this? What will happen to you?'

Client: 'I will be all alone in these big houses and there will be no one to love me.'

Vianna: 'Would you like to know what it feels like to have someone there with you?'

Client: 'It's impossible. I'm not lovable. No one wants to share this with me.'

These are the main issues that are keeping this person from obtaining their goals. With permission, the feelings and programmes of 'I am lovable' and 'It's possible to share a dream with another person' are downloaded.

Now the client is more nervous than before.

Vianna: 'What's wrong?'

Client: 'If I come together with someone, they'll find out who I really am! They won't want to be with me if they find out who I really am!'

Vianna: 'Well, who are you *really?*'

Client: 'I don't know. But they wouldn't like me if they saw me for who I really was.'

Vianna: 'Who told you this? Where did you first hear this?'

Client: 'I'm not sure, but I think that it was my mother. She told me that I'd never have anyone to love me and that I'd never amount to anything.'

These last statements are the bottom beliefs. These are the programmes that will be pulled, cancelled, resolved, sent to the Creator of All That Is and replaced with the correct programmes.

I will also ask the client if they want to receive the downloads of 'I am lovable', 'I can be respected' and 'There is someone out there for me'. If they do not receive these downloads, their incredibly brilliant brain (that is creating the life that they truly want) will not change on a subconscious level. If the subconscious level changes, the client can manifest what they want.

The mind is amazing. We actually create what our subconscious mind believes to be reality. If we say that we *have no money* and that we are *barely making it*, the subconscious will take this as an order or a demand and create what it thinks we want. These are some of the first things that you look for in a belief work session as you dig for the bottom belief.

It is important for the client to know that it is not only *possible* to be loved and to be healthy, but that these are *obtainable*. Some of the downloads to make sure that the client accepts this will pertain to *goals* downloads such as 'I can obtain my goals', 'I know how to set up a goal' and 'I know how to plan' (*see page 239*). By themselves these downloads will make a big difference to a person's life.

DIGGING WORK EXAMPLE 5: THE EGYPTIAN GODDESS

The Creator told me to pull up a specific person as a demonstration in one of my teachers' certification classes in Yellowstone, Montana. She was a beautiful, tall African-American woman in a white dress, and looked and moved as though she were an Egyptian goddess. I silently said to myself, 'Creator, you have made a mistake. This woman is perfect. Obviously, you need to give me someone who has more troubles to work on.' But the Creator insisted that I bring her to the middle to work with her as a class example.

Vianna: 'What would you like to work on?'

Woman: 'I'm afraid of being a healer. I think it's from a past life.'

You should know that this kind of statement can be the result of sexual abuse, or abuse of any kind. The person will try to pretend the issue is from a past life because they don't want to deal with it in this life. It is possible that it is from a past life, but if they make a statement like this, it's probably from this life.

Vianna: 'Why are you afraid of being a healer?'

Woman: 'Because I might die.'

At this point I heard the Creator say to me, 'Ask her why she had to hide when she was a child.'

Vianna: 'Why did you have to hide as a child?'

Woman: 'I had to hide to sneak food to my brother and sisters.'

After this statement, the story came pouring out of her. Her mother had died, leaving her and three other small children, one of whom was a two-year-old girl. Her father had taken them to an aunt and uncle who hadn't fed them properly. They were all malnourished, particularly the youngest girl. When the father remarried he came to get them, but the same thing happened again with their stepmother – she would not feed the children properly, particularly the small girl. The family would eat food in front of her and she would be forced to sit still and watch them. The woman told me she had been severely beaten for sneaking out and trying to get food from the cupboard to feed the others. From that time on, she always felt that she had to hide.

One day, the two-year-old girl didn't get up because she had starved to death. Her stepmother kicked her across the room to try to wake her up. Then she put her in my client's arms and drove to the hospital. The hospital staff immediately saw that the girl had starved to death and the other children were malnourished. They took them all away from the parents and put them in foster homes.

I was told to tell the woman that her little sister had given her life so that she and the other two children might live. I told her that we were going to clear her sorrow from the past.

When she had first sat down in front of me, I hadn't dreamed that she had gone through all that abuse; I hadn't seen it because she was so confident. Before you make judgements about people, you should know that some of the worst cases of abuse are the people who seem absolutely together. Abused people are the best fakers and usually the best at hiding their pain. They are the ones who always smile and laugh. But it is a fake laugh. They seem present, but they're not really there. You can see it in their eyes and what is behind them. Yet they smile self-assuredly because they don't want you to know that they are hurting inside. They often develop intestinal problems.

With issues of abuse, you have to stay persistent and make sure that the person knows they are loved.

Teaching this woman what it felt like to be safe cleared her of issues around being a healer, but more belief work was necessary.

DIGGING WORK EXAMPLE 6: FATHER ISSUES

Vianna: 'What would you like the final outcome of this session to be for you? What do you want to do with your life? If there were anything you would like to change, what would it be?'

Young woman: 'I would like to get over the feeling that I'm never good enough.'

Vianna: 'Who taught you that feeling?'

Young woman: 'It was my father. I resent him because he taught me that I was only a seven.'

Vianna: 'What does that mean?'

Young woman: 'What that means is that on a scale of one to ten I'm a little bit better than average, but I'll never be good enough. I am only a seven and I'll never be a ten.'

Vianna: 'Did you believe him when he told you this?'

Young woman: 'Yes, I believed him. I don't know why I believed him. I deeply resent him now.'

Vianna: 'Why do you resent him?'

Young woman: 'Because he made me feel terrible about myself.'

Vianna: 'How did he do this?'

Young woman: 'He just said things like that.'

Vianna: 'How did this help you in your life? How did it serve you?'

Young woman: 'I learned that I could never get enough, do enough or be enough, so I might as well settle for less.'

Vianna: 'Have you settled for less all your life?'

Young woman: 'Yes, I have. All my life I've settled for less.'

Vianna: 'This almost sounds like an excuse so that you don't have to apply yourself to get the best that life has to offer.'

Young woman: 'I guess so. I guess I could thank my father for that. I won't have to try as long as I don't think I can do it.'

Vianna: 'What would happen if you were to try?'

Young woman: 'I would fail.'

Vianna: 'What would happen if you failed?'

Young woman: 'I'd have to settle for less.'

Vianna: 'What would happen if you succeeded?'

Young woman: 'I don't know what would happen if I succeeded. I have no idea. I guess it's better to fail and know what happens than to succeed and not know the outcome.'

Vianna: 'So really you are afraid to succeed.'

Young woman: 'I guess so. I've never thought of it like that. I guess as long as I resent my father I won't have to succeed.'

Vianna: 'So it's easier to resent your father than to discover the unknown.'

Young woman: 'I guess so.'

Vianna: 'Would you like to know what it feels like to live without fear of the unknown? What it feels like to know how to take the next step, to know that it's possible?'

Young woman: 'Yes! Yes, I would.'

By instilling these feeling downloads, the programme of 'I am only a seven' is cleared. Now we use the energy testing. With the client holding her fingers firmly together, I have her say, 'I am only a seven.' Sure enough, this belief is cleared.

Then I energy-test for the programme of 'I resent my father'. This too is cleared. The realization that it was safer to resent her father than it was to succeed has permitted her 'computer mind' to move forward. The feeling downloads have helped her to move forward in a smooth transition.

This is digging work at its best. With this work, you find not only the most negative and sorrowful belief, but also how it is serving that person.

If you don't follow through to the bottom belief, you will only partially clear the issues. I'm sure that there are many people who have left a belief work session only partially cleared of their issues. Still, it is better to be partially cleared than not cleared at all. On some level these people will have improved, but nothing compares to the peace of mind of finding the bottom belief.

DIGGING WORK EXAMPLE 7: HEALING

Vianna: 'What is the outcome you want from this session?'

Hiro Myiazaki: 'I want to manifest a great healing practice, to have the people who come to me heal all the time, to have lots of money, lots of time and a happy family.'

Vianna: 'OK, imagine that all this is yours. Imagine that people are coming to you from everywhere to be healed. How does this make you feel?'

Hiro: 'Good. This makes me feel fine.'

Vianna: 'Can you handle all these hundreds of people coming to you to be healed?'

Hiro: 'Of course. I know how to set my boundaries.'

Vianna: 'I want you to imagine that you are living this situation. What does it feel like?'

Hiro: 'Well ... I feel that eventually I will fail, that I will mess up working on someone.'

This is a early indication that there is a bottom belief that will block this man from succeeding as a healer.

Vianna: 'What would happen if you messed up?'

Hiro: 'Oh, they would cast me away. They would put me in a hole.'

Vianna: 'A hole?'

Hiro: 'Yes, a black hole and they would forget about me.'

Vianna: 'What happens to you in this hole?'

Hiro: 'Nothing happens to me. They have forgotten about me.'

Vianna: 'How long will they forget about you?'

Hiro: 'I don't know. Forever maybe, because I messed up. I hurt someone and they got sick because of my healing. Because of this I got pushed away.'

Vianna: 'Will you ever be forgiven?'

Hiro: 'No, I will never be forgiven.'

Vianna: 'So what happens?'

Hiro: 'I can't stand the loneliness. I find a sharp object and I commit suicide.'

Vianna: 'Are you free of this experience now? Do you go to the light? What happens to you?'

Hiro: 'I'm in the darkness and I'm afraid to come out. I'm afraid to fail again.'

Vianna: 'How long are you in the darkness?'

Hiro: 'I'm not sure. Five thousand years comes to my mind.'

Vianna: 'Then what happens to you?'

Hiro: 'I go to the light. I am given another chance.'

Vianna: 'So really, what is the ultimate fear associated with you doing healing work?'

Hiro: 'That I will fail. That it will be my fault and I will be pushed away. I will be alone, cast out and forgotten.'

Vianna to class: 'These are the bottom beliefs. The reason Hiro cannot realize his true life's ambition is because of the fear of obtaining it. Therefore, if you pull and release the programmes of "I am afraid I will be alone" and "I will be forgotten", they should be replaced with "I know what it feels like to be remembered", "I know how to live and have someone there", "I know how to forgive myself", "I know that the Creator is the healer" and "It's safe to be a healer".'

Vianna to Hiro: 'Do I have permission to release these programmes and replace them as I have suggested?'

Hiro: 'Yes. Thank you very much!'

Hiro leaves the belief work session shiny, light and full of joy.

DIGGING WORK EXAMPLE 8:
INTUITION AND PSYCHIC ABILITIES

Vianna: 'Do I have permission to enter your space?'

Woman: 'Yes, you do.'

Vianna: 'How old are you?'

Woman: 'Fifty-three years old.'

Vianna: 'Do you have any questions?'

Woman: 'I want to know how to open up and be more intuitive.'

Vianna to class: 'OK, so that is where we are going to start. Don't start with what *you* think a person needs. Start with what *they* think they need. The client's request is number one.'

Vianna to woman: 'Repeat after me: "I know how to open up and be more intuitive."'

Woman: 'I know how to open up and be more intuitive. I know I am intuitive. I know I can control my intuition.'

Vianna to class: 'OK, she has energy-tested negative for these programmes. She wants to open up, but she doesn't think she can control it.'

Vianna to woman: 'Why can't you open up intuitively?'

Woman: 'Because I am afraid.'

Vianna: 'Why are you afraid?'

Woman: 'I am afraid of what will happen to me. I am afraid that I will change so much I won't know who I am. I am afraid that this will happen gradually, over time, and I won't know that it is happening.'

Vianna: 'If you change so much that you won't know who you are, what will happen then?'

Woman: 'I will lose myself.'

Vianna: 'And that means *what* to you? Repeat after me: "I am afraid to lose myself."'

Woman: 'I am afraid to lose myself.'

She energy tests 'Yes.'

Vianna: 'Why are you lost?'

Woman: 'I am afraid I will find myself.'

Vianna: 'What will happen if you find yourself?'

Woman: 'I am afraid that if I find myself I will find my life's mission, and I am afraid I will fail in my mission in this life. What if it makes me do something I don't want to do?'

Vianna: 'Repeat after me: "I am afraid of my life's mission."'

Woman: 'I am afraid of my life's mission.'

She energy-tests 'Yes.'

Vianna: 'What's the worst thing that would happen if you started your life's work?'

Woman: 'I am afraid it would tarnish my reputation. I am afraid I would fail at it.'

Vianna to class: 'Now, did I put those words in her mouth? No, I went up and asked God. The Creator said, "She is afraid she will fail." This is likely to be the bottom issue. If I start pulling all the other beliefs that she has along the way, the session is going to take a long time and it's not going to get to the bottom issue. So let's go with this one. You will notice that I am touching her hand while I am working with her. This is to comfort her and hold her space for her.'

Vianna to woman: 'If you had a fear every day, what would it be?'

Woman: 'I would be afraid of the people that I worked on and tried to heal.'

Vianna: 'Are you are afraid you will fail them?'

Woman: 'Yes, I am afraid I will fail the people I am working on. I am afraid I will fail God. I am afraid I will fail myself.'

Vianna to class: 'If she energy-tests positive for failing the people she is working on and negative for failing God, what does that tell me? It tells me that she is afraid of failing the people she is working on. There might be some God issues in there somewhere that we may bring up, but she is actually afraid she will hurt the people.'

Woman: 'I am afraid I will kill them. I am afraid I will hurt them. I am afraid I will fail them.'

Vianna to class: 'She is definitely concerned for them!'

Vianna to woman: 'What's the worst thing that would happen if you failed them?'

Woman: 'It would be devastating.'

Vianna: 'Why?'

Woman: 'I would be letting them down.'

Vianna: 'If you let them down, what would happen?'

Woman: 'I don't know. I would be killed.'

Vianna to class: 'OK, so does she have a fear of dying? Or is her big fear of hurting others. Could it be that simple?'

Vianna to woman: 'So, should we teach you what it feels like to do healings without hurting others and to know what you are doing? Let us teach you *to know what to do and how to help people. How to connect with God and know what to do in healings. How to live without the fear of failing those people and how to know that it is possible. How to know what it feels like to know that everyone you work with actually receives a healing.* Do you accept these energies?'

Woman: 'Yes.'

Vianna to woman: 'Since God does the healings, does God let those people down? Say, "I am afraid that God will let those people down."'

Woman: 'I am afraid that God will let me down.'

She energy-tests 'Yes.'

Vianna: 'Why?'

Woman: 'I don't deserve it.'

Vianna: 'You say you don't deserve to ask God these things. What makes you feel that way? What if God doesn't listen to you one day?'

Woman: 'Then nothing happens.'

Vianna to woman: 'To trust that God will heal these people is a big step for you. Would you like to know how to take that step? Would you accept these downloads:

"I know what to do when someone is ill."

"I know how to help people."

"I know how to be a healer."

'Would you like to know how to live without the fear that God will let you down and that you will let those people down? Do you accept these energies?'

Woman: 'Yes.'

Vianna: 'Good. How do you feel now?'

Woman: 'Much better!'

Vianna to class: 'You see, she didn't know how to take the next step or how to heal another person. She didn't know how to trust the Creator completely.'

Vianna to woman: 'Would you like to know how to take the next step? Do I have permission to download you with this knowledge, and the knowledge that it's possible and that you deserve it and are worthy of it? Do you accept these energies?'

Woman: 'Yes.'

Vianna: 'How do you feel now?'

Woman: 'I feel a slight shift.'

Vianna: 'Would you like a bigger shift? Would you like to know how to work on somebody without feeling performance anxiety? Would you like to know how to be patient with yourself? To allow your mind, your body and your spirit to learn effortlessly? Let's teach you when to know that you have completed working on yourself and when your body is tired. When to rest and when to honour what your body says and also when to honour what you are here to do. Do you accept these energies?'

Woman: 'Yes.'

Vianna to class: 'So she is finished and the bottom issue was that she was really afraid of hurting others. We didn't go any deeper than that. She really has a natural concern for others. Now she is going to be more confident.'

Vianna to woman in conclusion: 'Do I have permission to teach you how to listen to your heart and to the Creator? To know when to make a decision and how to make a decision? To know what to tell your clients without hurting them?'

Woman: 'Yes.'

Listening is one of the most important things in belief work. Too often the practitioner will attempt to tell the person what *they* believe their beliefs are. *Listening to the client and to the Creator is an art – an art that takes practice.* The reason for this is that all the messages that you get from the Creator have to be interpreted by your mind. And you have to be sure that the message that you receive from the Creator and the one that you give the person are exactly the same.

DIGGING WORK EXAMPLE 9: WEAKER PEOPLE TAKE ADVANTAGE

Vianna to class: 'One of the first questions that I ask a person before I start a reading pertains to any drugs and herbs that they might be taking. The reason that I ask this before I look into their body is so that I don't become confused by the essences of the compounds that I will come into contact with in the reading. Any drug or herb changes a person's vibration, and the way it is interacting with the body can mask their disease or disorder. Once you have experienced what drugs and herbs feel like in the body, it will be easy to recognize them for what they are when you are in a reading. But to save valuable time, I ask the person what they are taking before I go into the body.'

Vianna to woman: 'Are you taking any drugs or herbs? Did you take magnesium this morning or any vitamins?'

Woman: 'No.'

Vianna: 'The next thing I do as I enter into the body is to say to the Creator, "Creator, show me!" So I see that this woman grinds her teeth because of parasites. There are parasites in the colon. I see that she is in love. If you pass through the energy of a person's heart, you will find out whether they are in love or not. I see her spine is out of alignment. Do you want the Creator to straighten up your back?'

Woman: 'Yes, please!'

Vianna: 'You have met huge challenges in your life and I can see that you're ready for joy. Your knees are weak, you're scared to move on in your life and you should know that it will be OK. In the past, you were inundated by heavy metals, but now, little by little, the magnesium you are using is flushing them from your system. The hearing in one of your ears is better than in the other. Has it always been like that?'

Woman: 'It was an accident that caused slight hearing loss.'

Vianna: 'What comes into your mind if you hear the word "parasite"?'

Woman: 'My father.'

Vianna: 'Is your mother alive?'

Woman: 'No, she's not. I am adopted.'

Vianna: 'Tell me about your adoptive father.'

Woman: 'Both my adoptive parents are parasites.'

Vianna: 'Why do you allow them to behave that way?'

Woman: 'I don't know how to change things.'

Vianna: 'Will you allow me to teach you how to say "no" in life and to say "no" to them?'

Woman: 'Yes, I accept these downloads.'

Vianna: 'Now that you are able to answer with a "no" to them, what will happen to you? What is the first thing that comes into your mind?'

Woman: 'I think that they are weak.'

Vianna: 'I know. Do you feel you must help them because they're weaker than you? Say: "I must allow weaker people to take advantage of me."'

Woman: 'I must allow weaker people to take advantage of me.'

She energy-tests 'Yes.'

Vianna: 'Say: "I must let stronger people take advantage of me."'

Woman: 'I must let stronger people take advantage of me.'

She energy-tests 'No.'

Vianna: 'Only weaker people take advantage of you. Why?'

Woman: 'I have to help them.'

Vianna: 'Do you have to help those who are weaker than you even if they're hurting you in some way? You're not able to say "no" because they're weaker than you. So you let them take advantage of you without teaching them how to be stronger. What's the worst thing that would happen to you if you didn't help them? Would you feel guilty?'

Woman: 'I would feel bad and I would lose my self-esteem.'

Vianna: 'Repeat after me: "I have self-esteem."'

The woman energy-tests 'Yes.'

Vianna: 'Why do you underestimate yourself?'

Woman: 'I don't think I deserve this life. I don't deserve to exist.'

Vianna: 'Repeat after me: "I exist."'

The woman energy-tests 'No.'

Vianna: 'Would you like to have the Creator's definition of existing?'

Woman: 'Yes.'

Vianna: 'Did your adoptive parents destroy your feeling of existing? Who made you feel this way?

Woman: 'I don't know.'

Vianna: 'Would you like the feeling that you have your own place in the world and you have value and can shine? Will you permit me to teach you how to love your parents without feeling drained and how to receive and accept love?'

Woman: 'Yes.'

Vianna: 'Now you can love your adoptive parents without feeling drained by them. How do you feel now? Better? Does your body hurt anywhere?'

Woman: 'My stomach aches.'

Vianna: 'What other kind of pain do you feel?'

Woman: 'A dull pain in the solar plexus.'

Vianna: 'Do you feel lonely as well?'

Woman: 'Yes, I do.'

Vianna: 'Stomach disorders are linked to shame, distress and feelings of guilt. Would you like to be able to say "no" in life when you need to feel confident and live without being abused?'

Woman: 'Yes.'

Vianna: 'How do you feel now?'

Woman: 'The pain has gone from my stomach but it has moved.'

Vianna: 'Where has it moved to?'

Woman: 'My legs and my arms...'

Vianna to class: 'As you pick on up problems and eliminate them, they can move somewhere else in the body. As you release something, you always have to ask if another part of the body aches. You can ask the Creator where the pain is, but also ask the person you're working with.'

Woman: 'My bones ache now.'

Vianna: 'This is very important. The aching in different parts of the body means that the emotions attached to that area have been stimulated. Maybe you feel violated and you wonder why nobody protected you. Have you ever felt protected by anyone?'

Woman: 'Nobody but myself.'

Vianna: 'Would you allow me to teach you how to feel protected, how to protect yourself and how to let someone else protect you?'

Woman: 'Yes.'

Vianna to class: 'These aren't programmes that I am releasing and replacing, it's about teaching her feelings and knowing from the Creator of All That Is.'

Vianna to woman: 'How do you feel now? Is the pain still there?'

Woman: 'Yes, it is.'

Vianna: 'Why is it still hurting?'

Woman: 'Because of the other people who have hurt me.'

Vianna: Repeat after me: "I let weaker people hurt me." *[She energy-tests "Yes."]* Can I teach you that you don't have to let weaker people hurt you and the right way to deal with these situations?'

Woman: 'Yes. The pain is getting worse now.'

Vianna: 'Where was God in your life when you were young?'

Woman: 'God betrayed me.'

Vianna: 'Repeat after me: "God betrayed me." *[She energy-tests "Yes."]* I could go on digging, but I know the problem is in the bones. You are convinced that God betrayed you and so God doesn't exist. There's a contradiction in your body. Am I allowed to teach you how to have expectations of God and to know that people will understand you?'

Woman: 'Yes.'

Vianna: 'You have the programme of "I allow the people I love to hurt me". Can I release this? Am I allowed to teach you that there is love without pain, that you are able to love and you know the right definition of God?'

Woman: 'Yes. Now my right hip aches.'

Vianna to class: 'Some moments ago the pain was in the left part. This can mean that she was abused when she was young, or maybe that somebody told her she was ugly or bad or something.'

Vianna to woman: 'Touch your right hip. What do you feel?'

Woman: 'I feel sick to my stomach.'

Vianna: 'Don't vomit now. It's almost over. Do you want to know that you are safe?'

Woman: 'Yes.'

Vianna: 'Touch your stomach. What do you feel?'

Woman: 'I want to disappear.'

Vianna: 'Do I have permission to teach you how to live each day without feeling abandoned, to know that it is safe to be here and to know how to live without wanting to disappear? Do I have permission to work on the time when you were still a foetus in your mother's womb?'

Woman: 'Yes, you can.'

Vianna: 'How do you feel now?'

Woman: 'My back aches.'

Vianna: 'What do you know about your true parents?'

Woman: 'Nothing.'

Vianna: 'Do I have permission give you the feeling of what it feels to be loved by your real mother and father from the womb?'

Woman: 'Yes.'

Vianna: 'How do you feel now?'

Woman: 'My back still aches. I feel calmer, but there's still something wrong in my knees and in my legs.'

Vianna to class: 'On an emotional level, she's quiet, but her body continues to ache. This is called disassociation. She has learned to switch her emotions off when they get to be too much. Healers are often able to disassociate.'

Vianna to woman: 'Do I have permission to teach you that it's safe to feel emotions?'

Woman: 'Yes.'

Vianna to woman: 'What are you feeling now?'

Woman: 'My legs hurt.'

Vianna: 'The energy has moved to the legs, which are the support of the body. What is the worst thing that can happen to you if you are loved simply for who you are?'

Woman: 'I don't know. It's something I've never known.'

Vianna: 'Repeat after me: "I know what being loved for who I am means."'

The woman energy-tests 'No.'

Vianna to class: 'I taught her how to accept love from her parents, but her body is not able to integrate these feelings. It's easier for her to accept the pain than to be open for love, because she understands suffering better. She needs magnesium and calcium. If you're not able to accept love, you're not able to accept magnesium and calcium. Do I have permission to teach you how to feel loved just because of who you are?'

Woman: 'Yes.'

Vianna: 'How is the pain now?'

Woman: 'It's strong at the juncture between hip and femur.'

Vianna: 'Repeat after me: "I know how to live without pain." *[She energy-tests "No."]* Do I have permission to teach you this feeling?'

Woman: 'Yes.'

Vianna: 'How is the pain now?'

Woman: 'It is beginning to fade. It is gone now.'

Vianna: 'Her body looks refreshed and she is much lighter.'

DIGGING WORK EXAMPLE 10: ABUNDANCE

Vianna: 'What would you like to work on?'

Woman: 'On abundance. ThetaHealing has helped me to come out of a difficult situation that ended in divorce. But because of that, I have financial problems.'

Vianna: 'Abundance can be reached in many ways.'

Woman: 'Yes, but I haven't been helped. Nobody has given me anything.'

Vianna: 'OK, but I have my own ideas on abundance. What does abundance mean to you?'

Woman: 'I want to be free and independent of other people.'

Vianna: 'And what if God thinks that it would be right for you to have a partner as well?'

Woman: 'That would be OK, but I want to be economically independent.'

Vianna: 'Being helped by someone else does not mean being dependent. I think that you have programmes about God and money. What is the worst thing that could happen if you had a lot of money?'

Woman: 'I wouldn't know how to handle it.'

Vianna: 'Let's teach you how to deal with a lot of money. Imagine you are rich. What are you going to do?'

Woman: 'I can do and have whatever I want – books, culture, seminars, travelling, no more problems...'

Vianna: 'And what would you do without problems?'

Woman: 'I would have fun. I would enjoy life.'

Vianna: 'And then?'

Woman: 'I would help other people.'

Vianna: 'Who?'

Woman: 'Those who need help.. My family, my relatives..'

Vianna: 'OK, and what would happen next?'

Woman: 'I don't know.'

Vianna: 'And if you knew what would happen next?'

Woman: 'I wouldn't have problems paying bills.'

Vianna: 'But which problems would you have if those you listed before disappeared?'

Woman: 'None! Except those from my children.'

Vianna: 'What would happen if you were to help your children too much?'

Woman: 'They would take advantage of me. Everybody would pretend they loved me.'

Vianna: 'How would you know who really loved you?'

Woman: 'Maybe nobody would really love me.'

Vianna: 'So have you always been the one who cared about everybody?'

Woman: 'I've always given a lot and received little back. So if I have abundance, the people in my life will want more. They will spoil my life.'

Vianna: 'So would you say that abundance would spoil your life somehow?'

Woman: 'I'm not sure I've ever had abundance in my life.'

Vianna: 'Repeat after me: "I'm afraid of abundance."'

The woman energy-tests 'Yes.'

Vianna: 'Repeat after me: "If I have too much money and abundance, people will exploit me and will love me just because of what I can give them." *[She energy-tests "Yes" again.]* So you would like to be rich?'

Woman: 'Yes, but I'm afraid of being rich.'

Vianna: 'OK. Do I have permission to teach you how to live without being scared of having a lot of money and without letting other people, especially those you love, take advantage of you? Do you want to learn how to feel loved and helped without losing your freedom?'

Woman: 'Yes.'

Vianna: 'What is the worst thing about having a lot of money?'

Woman: 'Nothing.'

Vianna: 'Do you like teaching at seminars?'

Woman: 'Yes, but I've never led one. I'd like to use Theta not only for seminars, but also for other things such as improving my mind's faculties and helping other people and myself.'

Vianna: 'Do you want the advantages that abundance gives you?'

Woman: 'Yes!'

Vianna: 'Repeat after me: "Healers need to be poor." *[She energy-tests 'Yes."]* Why do you feel that healers need to be poor?'

Woman: 'I don't know. Maybe because you know what suffering means if you have been poor.'

Vianna: 'You are convinced that to be a healer you have to suffer, aren't you? *[She energy-tests 'Yes."]* Would you like to know that you've already suffered enough and you can go forward without being poor? Do you think you have gained the right to experience abundance? *[She energy-tests 'No."]* What do you have to do to reach abundance?'

Woman: 'I think I have cleared my faults and my debts. I think I have the right to have abundance.'

Vianna: 'Let's see if you regain your privileges to abundance by this Friday.'

Woman: 'Great! Now I will have to play the Super-lotto!'

Vianna: 'What if by Friday you gain your rights back once and for all? What then?'

Woman: 'I don't know.'

Vianna: 'Let's teach you that there's a solution for every situation and how to recognize it:

"I will recognize the solution when I see it."

"I believe that God will take care of me."

"I free the people around me from the programme that they must disappoint me."

"I can trust the thought that God will take care of me."

"I am given solutions to improve my life."

'Do I have permission to give you these downloads?'

Woman: 'Yes.'

Vianna to class: 'Observe her – she's very quiet now. The only thing that made her nervous was the idea of trusting God. That's our starting-point for digging for the bottom belief. It could be about men and not about God...'

Vianna to woman: 'Who disappointed you?'

Woman: 'Everybody.'

Vianna: 'Why?'

Woman: 'Because they took advantage of me. They took everything from me because I was generous. I'm still generous – I'm always giving and I never receive anything back.'

Vianna to class: 'I can see from her reactions that this is the right direction.'

Vianna to woman: 'Your heart is very sad. What do you do when people behave this way towards you?'

Woman: 'I get angry. But if my children take advantage of me, I don't manage to say "no".'

Vianna: 'Are you able to say "no" to the people you love?'

Woman: 'Maybe not.'

Vianna: 'Do you know how to receive love from your children?'

Woman: 'I'm starting to doubt it.'

Vianna: 'What do your children give you back?'

Woman: 'They love me, but I recognize they are selfish. Anyway, I've been disappointed by everybody, not only by my children.'

Vianna: 'Do your parents love you?'

Woman: 'I've never felt loved by them and now my father is dead.'

Vianna: 'Why didn't you feel loved by him?'

Woman: 'Because I can't remember being happy with him.'

Vianna: 'Tell me more.'

Woman: 'My mother has always preferred my brother over me. I feel that I am never enough.'

Vianna: 'Repeat after me: "I'm never enough." *[She energy-tests 'Yes.'']* Do you want to know how to live day after day feeling you're enough and knowing how it feels to be loved, knowing you're enough?

Woman: 'Yes.'

Vianna to class: 'I went up to the Creator and asked what I should insert. I know that it's easier for her to let her children disappoint her than receive love back. I taught her how to feel that she is enough. Her children love her deeply. She can have abundance without feeling lonely. I also inserted a new definition of the Creator and the concept that one can receive love and at the same time be free.'

Vianna to woman: 'How do you feel now?'

Woman: 'Fine...'

Vianna: 'But...?'

Woman: 'I feel I have lost something.'

Vianna: 'What do you feel you have lost?'

Woman: 'I don't know. Maybe it's the idea that I haven't really paid for everything bad I've done during my past lives. I have the feeling that I still have some debts and bills to pay from past lives that will soon come due.'

Vianna: 'Would you like to know how it feels to live without debts?'

Woman: 'Yes. I feel I'm too complicated.'

Vianna: 'What about?'

Woman: 'Well, the way that I am.'

Vianna: 'But women *are* complicated! It's the characteristic that makes us women and the thing that confuses men.'

Woman: 'There's a rage in my heart.'

Vianna: 'Why? What or who makes you feel this way?'

Woman: 'I don't know, it's nothing in particular. It's just the fact that I work hard, I get to a certain point and then something comes along and spoils everything.'

Vianna: 'Do I have permission to teach you the feeling of having a plan that gets realized easily and successfully, the knowledge of what a good plan is, the intuition to understand if it will work and the feeling of taking action and arriving at the end?'

Woman: 'Yes.'

Vianna: 'Repeat after me: "I have to fail in order to make my mother happy. I'm afraid of being successful." *[She energy-tests "Yes" to both.]* Do I have permission to give you the feeling of how to live without being scared by success? Let's teach you how to accept the success you deserve and how to recognize it.'

Woman: 'Yes.'

Vianna to class: 'She is almost finished, but she still needs something else... She may need the programmes of:

"I have to accept myself."

"I am enough for myself."

"I feel grateful for my life."

"I feel excited about life."

"Life is an adventure and life has romance."

"I know how to open my heart to the pleasure of living."'

Vianna to woman: 'Do I have permission to teach you how to permit money to come into your life? To have the pleasure of loving and being loved by the people around you? Of letting the barriers you have made to keep them out fall down? Of having the freedom of being emotional and permitting your soul mate to come into your life?'

Woman: 'Yes.'

Vianna to class: 'Is she ready to receive abundance now? She has accepted that her life can follow that path, so we will wait and see. I have explored to see whether she knows that abundance will come or fears it coming too easily. If we feel that things are too easy, we may feel that we don't deserve them. But now I have given her the knowledge that abundance can come easily, she won't feel strange when it does come.

'We are finished with this session and I can see that she is OK, just a bit nervous... Knowing that your life is going to change radically always generates new emotions.

'In a belief work session, you have to be attentive to what the Creator tells you. You can't simply listen to what your client is telling you. You also have to go up to the Creator and ask what the person needs.'

DIGGING WORK EXAMPLE 11: **DIABETES**

This session was with a woman in an Intuitive Anatomy class.

Vianna: 'What would you like to work on?'

Woman: 'My diabetes. It came on when my father died. I was very sad and angry because I hadn't seen him in years. I went to Brazil to spend two months with him so that we could have closure about the past. I knew he was afraid because he knew he had to explain certain things to me about why he had treated me and my siblings the way he did. I wanted to know what he had to tell me, but he died before I could talk to him. When he died, he was 72 years old and had no health problems. Suddenly he had a heart attack and died without having the chance to talk to me. I felt so bad about all this.

'Then the doctors told me I had diabetes. Because of the neuropathies, I suffer from insensitivity in the legs. I can't feel my feet and I have problems with balance. I have to take insulin – I take it four times a day, before meals and before going to sleep – and I keep putting on weight.'

Vianna: 'Do you feel defeated by your father? Do you think he won because he managed to avoid talking to you? Repeat after me:

"I feel discouraged."

"Diabetes cannot be cured."

"I'm a warrior."

"Diabetes weakens me."

"Diabetes is defeating me."'

She energy tests "Yes" to all of them.

Vianna: 'How do you feel when you say those things?'

Woman: 'I don't know. Some of them don't pass though my brain as thoughts, but I can feel some of them.'

Vianna: 'Is there still something to resolve between you and your father?'

Woman: 'Yes. He doesn't know everything I wanted to tell him.'

Vianna: 'How do you feel about it?'

Woman: 'Disappointed. It was very important to me to tell him how I felt.'

Vianna: 'What would you tell him if you could?'

Woman: 'That he wasn't a good father and he wasn't able to love people in general. He was selfish and self-centred. I was angry with him because he hurt me and my brothers.'

Vianna: 'We will work on your rage about your father. Because it lies in the liver, we will work there. We are going to melt the rage you feel towards your father. This rage was created to protect yourself from him. You feel defeated by the diabetes, so much so that you feel you want to stop living. Do I have permission to teach you that you haven't been defeated and you have the power to beat diabetes? Because this is what you were about to do when your father died: take your power back. Do I have your permission to do all this?'

Woman: 'Yes.'

Vianna: 'Do you want to forgive your father? Repeat after me: "I can forgive my father." *[She energy-tests 'No."]* What did this rage do for you?'

Woman: 'It gave me the strength to be different from him. He spent his life getting rich; I'm spending my energy helping people.'

Vianna: 'So this rage helped you to become the opposite of him. You used it to love other people. Would you like to continue on your path without being so angry? Are you ready to let this feeling go? Let's free your father from the obligation of making you angry with him. Would you like the feeling of "I know what it feels like to live without being angry with my father"? Do I have permission to insert this feeling?'

Woman: 'Yes.'

Vianna: 'If he is free from this obligation, you will be free as well. Sometimes the people that we think play a negative role in our life turn out to be positive for us. Now, I didn't instill how to forgive your father, or any other new programme, I simply freed you from the obligations that kept you in this conflict. Repeat after me: "I can forgive my father."'

Woman: 'I can forgive my father.'

She energy-tests 'Yes.'

Vianna: 'So you see, the programme has changed by itself through the insertion of a feeling. Whether you know it or not, this rage towards your father made you the beautiful person you are now. Since you had been treated badly by him, you made sure you treated everyone with respect. When I observe your pancreas and liver, I see that they are now working in a different way. Now perhaps you can permit your body to heal. Repeat after me: "I feel angry with my father" *[she energy-tests "No"]*, "I hate my father" *[she energy-tests "No"]*, "I can love my father" *[she energy-tests "Yes"]*. Do I have permission to teach your body how to gain nutrients from the food you eat?'

Woman: 'Yes.'

Vianna: 'Now you are free and can feel how much you miss your dad, instead of how much you hate him. It doesn't make him a better person in your eyes, but you can live in beauty now and can accept other people's help. There are probably more things to work on, but your sugar levels have gone down and now you will have to be careful about not going into hypoglycaemia. In the next few days you should monitor your sugars closely.'

Vianna to class: 'Never tell a client to stop taking insulin. Their doctor will do so when they see that their sugars are stabilizing.'

DIGGING WORK EXAMPLE 12: KIDNEYS

Vianna: 'Tell me about yourself.'

Man: 'I am a musician. I have always travelled and I have been one of the best at what I do. In 2000 I was in Brussels and one night I felt ill. I had just performed and I found I couldn't urinate. I went straight to hospital and they told me it was an inflammation, a kind of nephritis. The doctors told me, "Your kidneys are like two hard stones." They gave me antibiotics and something homoeopathic to maintain my recovery. Afterwards I felt quite good and continued to travel. Then last year, I was coming back from one of my tours and on the plane ride home I had another renal failure. I had to submit to dialysis. The symptoms were simple: I had to go to the toilet frequently, but I would only urinate a little. I'm still on dialysis.'

Vianna: 'OK, let's have a look at your organs. I don't know if the cause is bacterial or viral, but from its tone I think it's a virus. Has this problem made you stay at home more with your wife?'

Man: 'Yes.'

Vianna: 'Do you still travel a lot?'

Man: 'Yes. It's harder, but I still do it. I got ill in June, but I went to Italy in July and Cuba in August.'

Vianna: 'I feel that you want to stop travelling. Is this true?'

Man: 'Yes, it's a wish I have had for a long time because I've been around the world now and I get tired always being on the move.'

Vianna: 'This makes me wonder if you are ready for a healing. I feel that you are in love and you want to stop travelling in order to stay with your wife and relax. When you aren't with her you feel as if you're a fish out of water, don't you?'

Man: 'Because of my illness I feel safer at home than travelling around.'

Vianna: 'What would be the worst thing that would happen to you if you were to heal?'

Man: 'I can't imagine what the worst thing would be.'

Vianna: 'How would you feel if you went back to your music and your job?'

Man: 'Music is my life and passion, but I'd like to feel free to choose my own working schedule.'

Vianna: 'Are you forced to work a certain schedule?'

Man: 'I have been forced to travel for many years because I have had a lot of work contracts.'

Vianna: 'Can I teach you that you can be successful and at the same time spend as much time as you want with your wife?'

Man: 'Yes.'

Vianna: 'Why are you ill?'

Man: 'I've always performed, however tired I've been, and I've always been travelling. Then there are the vaccines I've had to take to travel to different countries... I think that there's a series of reasons.'

Vianna: 'This illness has made you realize that you have to relax more. The question is, can you maintain this relaxed feeling if you heal?'

Man: 'That's what I'd like, but I don't think I can.'

Vianna to class: 'Do you see the conflict?'

Vianna to man: 'Do I have permission to teach you that you can relax without getting ill and that you can live your passion but still be able to relax? Do you want to learn how to live without stress? To love your passion, your wife and yourself without feeling stressed?'

Man: 'Yes.'

Vianna: 'Repeat after me: "I'm ready to let this illness go." *[He energy-tests "Yes."]* "I have learned all the illness has to teach me." *[He energy-tests "Yes" again.]*'

Vianna to class: 'This belief work has helped him in many ways, but needs to be followed up by more sessions.'

Vianna to man: 'You are now free to accept a healing.'

DIGGING WORK EXAMPLE 13: ABUSE

Vianna: 'What would you like to work on?'

Woman: 'My father abused me from the age of four. He always scared me and I hated him. He always scared everybody – my mother, my sister, my brother and me. He always hurt me and if I told him to stop it, he got angry and locked me in my room. He abused me with words and beat me and my mother.'

Vianna: 'OK... What are your feelings towards him now?'

Woman: 'I don't hate him anymore, but I have had to work hard at it.'

Vianna: 'How do you feel about your mother?'

Woman: 'She tried to protect me, but it wasn't real protection because she didn't want to be hurt herself. I would watch her crying and pray to God to help her, because I loved her and I didn't want my father to kill her.'

Vianna: 'So are you angry with God?'

Woman: 'I don't feel that way.'

Vianna: 'Have you seen how her brain corrects things? She really worked on her feelings towards her father, but she feels she couldn't help her mother.'

Woman: 'I asked God to help her, but nothing happened. I didn't hate my father, I just felt really upset with him.'

Vianna: 'Red spots are appearing on your neck.'

Woman: 'Well, to this day he is abusing my mother. How would *you* feel?!'

Vianna: 'Can't you stop him? It seems you still feel powerless about the situation.'

Woman: 'Yes, and a thing that really hurt me was seeing my brother doing exactly the same thing with his son.'

Vianna: 'Repeat after me:

"I can't help my mother."

"Nobody can help my mother."

"Not even God can help my mother."'

The woman energy-tests 'Yes' to all.

Vianna: 'Why do you feel this way towards your mother?'

Woman: 'Because she lets him continue abusing her.'

Vianna: 'Do you accept this behaviour?'

Woman: 'No, I don't.'

Vianna: 'What does your mother say when you talk to her about it?'

Woman: 'She calls me two or three times a day to tell me how crazy my father is. For example, he gets mad if dinner isn't ready at the right time or if the potatoes aren't cooked the way they should be.'

Vianna: 'You said that life has been this way since you were four. What is the first thing you remember?'

Woman: 'He came back from work one day and looked angry. I was scared, so I hid in the closet. The only things I heard were my mother's screaming and my father's shouting.'

Vianna: 'Was that the first time you remember feeling so scared?'

Woman: 'Yes.'

Vianna: 'What else do you feel now, apart from powerless to help your mother?'

Woman: 'I feel trapped. Things are getting worse. When he's around other people, he behaves perfectly and they like him, but his mood changes when he comes home. I'm very angry about what he did in the past and continues to do now.'

Vianna: 'But you don't let him behave that way with you, do you?'

Woman: 'No. Now I manage to hug him when I go home to see my mother at Christmas.'

Vianna: 'Red spots appear on your skin when you talk about your mother.'

Woman: 'I feel sorry for her. She can't manage to leave him.'

Vianna: 'Tell me about their present life.'

Woman: 'He's angry all the time and I can't help her.'

Vianna: 'The way you speak about the situation it's as if you don't really feel it. Did your mother allow him to hurt you?'

Woman: 'She fears him. She says she simply wants to survive and won't get out of the situation.'

Vianna: 'Is this behaviour due to the way she was brought up?'

Woman: 'I don't know. I don't believe she's strong enough to leave.'

Vianna: 'Repeat after me:

> *"I have to be strong for my mother and myself."*
>
> *"I have to allow my father to hurt me so that he won't hurt my mother."*
>
> *"I'm my mother's mother."'*

The woman energy-tests 'Yes' to all.

Vianna: 'Do you know what being somebody's child means?'

Woman: 'No, I don't.'

Vianna: 'Have you ever been a small child?'

Woman: 'No, I haven't.'

Vianna: 'Repeat after me: "I have to hide from everything and everybody." *[She energy-tests "Yes."]* Have you ever felt safe?'

Woman: 'I feel safe now.'

Vianna: 'Do you know what safety at home means?'

Woman: 'No, I don't.'

Vianna: 'I'm a mother and as I touch your hand I realize that you have never felt loved as a daughter, never felt the warmth of a real home and have protected your own mother your whole life. Do I have permission to teach you what it feels like to be a child and live in a warm house and feel safe? This can have the same effect on your mother as well.'

Woman: 'Yes.'

Vianna: 'Repeat after me: "I can save my mother" *[she energy-tests "Yes"]*, "I must save my mother" *[she energy-tests "No"]*. You can't tell your mother to get out of the situation because she doesn't want to, but you can consider yourself out of it. Do you think she knows how a man is supposed to treat a woman in a normal relationship?'

Woman: 'No, she doesn't.'

Vianna: 'Why don't you tell her?'

Woman: 'She should know it already.'

Vianna: 'Is there any hope for your parents?'

Woman: 'No, there isn't.'

Vianna: 'You've lost hope for your mother.'

Woman: 'I've had to.'

Vianna: 'Why?'

Woman: 'Because she hasn't listened to me when I've tried to help her.'

Vianna: 'Has she ever listened to you?'

Woman: 'No, she hasn't.'

Vianna: 'Why?'

Woman: 'She doesn't want to.'

Vianna: 'Does she listen to anybody?'

Woman: 'No, she doesn't.'

Vianna: 'Do you get angry when somebody doesn't want to listen to you?'

Woman: 'Yes, I do.'

Vianna: 'Is your mother intelligent?'

Woman: 'No, she's not.'

Vianna: 'Repeat after me: "I hate my father." *[She energy-tests "Yes."]* Why is this belief still there? I thought you had released it. Repeat after me: "I hate what my father does to my mother. I hate my mother because she doesn't understand. I hate stupid people." *[She energy-tests "Yes" to all.]* What did you learn from your father?'

Woman: 'My father taught me that I don't have to tolerate such treatment. I am strong.'

Vianna: 'Your father taught you that you don't have to tolerate such treatment. Your mother didn't understand this message and you are angry with her for this reason. She managed to solve the question about your father with the idea that he has mental problems, but you are still frustrated by her reaction. What would you tell her if she could hear you?'

Woman: 'I'd tell her to leave him because he doesn't respect her. Does she like being treated that way?'

Vianna: 'Is she a victim? Are you angry with her because she simply accepts the situation?'

Woman: 'She **is** a victim. I told her to leave him, but she told me that she had to stay there. My father hates victims and so do I.'

Vianna: 'Repeat after me:

"My mother is weak."

"I hate victims."

"I hate people with no strength."

"I think they are ridiculous."

"I'll never be weak."

"I have to let weaker people take advantage of me."

"My mother is weak."

"My mother is a victim."

"My father is an abuser."'

The woman energy-tests 'Yes' to all.

Vianna: 'Do I have permission to teach you that weak people can't take advantage of you and that you can forgive them?'

Woman: 'Yes.'

Vianna: 'Repeat after me: "I have to save my mother. I can talk to my mother." *[She energy-tests "Yes" to both.]* Do I have permission to teach you how to live without tolerating abuse and how to live freely? This will help your mother, too, on a genetic level.'

Woman: 'Yes.'

Vianna: 'Because of your father, you are a strong woman. Repeat after me: "I'm a victim." *[She energy-tests "No".]* You don't hate your mother, but you are angry with her, with victims and with yourself. Thanks to these downloads, all these programmes have melted.'

Woman: 'When I was four years old, I shut the door in front of my father, I felt so scared.'

Vianna: 'Are you still feeling that fear?'

Woman: 'Yes, I am.'

Vianna: 'What is the worst thing that can happen if your father reaches you in the closet?'

Woman: 'He can beat me and shout at me.'

Vianna: 'Nothing worse?'

Woman: 'I can be forced to hate him.'

Vianna: 'And what happens if you hate him?'

Woman: 'When I was a child I wanted him dead.'

Vianna: 'What would have happened then, once he was dead?'

Woman: 'We would have known peace.'

Vianna: 'Repeat after me: "I know what it feels like to live in peace when my father is alive." *[She energy-tests "No."]* "I will know peace when my father is dead." *[She energy-tests "Yes."]* Do I have permission to change these programmes and download this feeling of peace?'

Woman: 'Yes.'

Vianna: 'When you were four, your father got angry with you because you shut the door in his face. How do you feel about it now?'

Woman: 'The fear has gone. I feel peaceful now.'

Vianna to class: 'She is light and happy now.'

DIGGING WORK EXAMPLE 14: **KEEPING A PROMISE**

Vianna: 'What would you like to work on?'

Man: 'An important part of my life has been erased because I was taken away from the land I was born in and I don't remember anything from that time. It's as if my roots have been cut. I was born in Australia and lately I feel a strong desire to go back there, but I don't know the reason for it.'

Vianna: 'So, what are you missing?'

Man: 'A friend of mine who lives there.'

Vianna: 'What's his name?'

Man: 'I don't know. I don't remember.'

Vianna: 'What did he look like when you last saw him?'

Man: 'He was a small child, an aborigine that I grew up with.'

Vianna: 'Who were his family?'

Man: 'I remember he had two sisters.'

Vianna: 'Well, you said you didn't remember anything from that time, but you remember many things! Did you promise him you would go back?'

Man: 'Yes, I did it before leaving.'

Vianna: 'And is your heart still communicating with that boy?'

Man: 'Yes, we keep in touch.'

Vianna: 'What does this mean to you?'

Man: 'I don't know. I think they're waiting for me.'

Vianna: 'Him and his family? How old would he be now?'

Man: 'He would be 45 or so.'

Vianna: 'When does he expect you to come back?'

Man: 'I didn't tell him how many years it would be.'

Vianna: 'But if you had said, what age would you have said?'

Man: 'Fifty. It's the first number that came into my mind.'

Vianna: 'Repeat after me: "I have agreed to go back when we are 50." *[He energy-tests "Yes."]* A soul fragment of that period stuck in your soul. Should we give it back to that time? Or do you want to keep this fragment? Do you want to go back?'

Man: 'Yes.'

Vianna: 'Repeat after me:

> *"I'm forced to fullfill my promise."*

> *"I want to fullfill it."*

> *"I have to go back to that country in order to regain my birthright."*

> *[He energy-tests "Yes" to all.]*

> *"I want my soul fragment back without going back to Australia."*

> *[He energy-tests "No."]*

'Do you get peace from this memory?'

Man: 'I get a sense of lightness from it.'

Vianna: 'Does it do you good, thinking of that period in time?'

Man: 'Yes, it does.'

Vianna: 'Can I ask the Creator to help you to recollect those memories easily?'

Man: 'Yes, you can.'

Vianna: 'What is your friend's name?'

Man: 'I think Ryan, but I'm not sure.'

Vianna: 'And his surname?'

Man: 'Something like Bramma.'

Vianna: 'Do you think you will find him if you go back?'

Man: 'Yes, I think so.'

Vianna: 'Do you know where you'll meet him?'

Man: 'Yes, I do.'

Vianna: 'Once you go back to Australia what will happen? Will you find your friend or will you be found by him?'

Man: 'I think we'll find each other.'

Vianna: 'I think you've already agreed on where and when to meet. Is your heart lighter now?'

Man: 'Yes, it is, but the pain has reached a higher area.'

Vianna: 'What are you feeling? What kind of pain is it?'

Man: 'It is a dull ache and I think it's the promise I made to go back.'

Vianna: 'Did your father force you to leave Australia?'

Man: 'Yes, he did. My sister and I tried everything we could to stay, but in the end we had to leave because my father had to see my grandfather, who was dying. Then we stayed in Italy. I don't know why we didn't move back to Australia.'

Vianna: 'Repeat after me: "I hate my father for bringing me here." *[He energy-tests "Yes."]* Do you want to release this feeling?'

Man: 'Yes, I do.'

Vianna: 'Repeat after me: "I hate my father for forcing me to leave Australia."'

He energy-tests 'No.'

Man: 'I can keep my promise to my friend.'

He energy-tests 'Yes.'

Vianna: 'Are you ready to work all around the world and have many houses in many countries?'

Man: 'Yes, I am.'

Vianna: 'I think you'll travel a lot. Are you married?'

Man: 'I have been married.'

Vianna: 'Has the pain in your upper chest disappeared?'

Man: 'It is lighter in the left part, but it persists in the right one.'

Vianna: 'It's from your father. Repeat after me: "I have to let my father hurt me." *[He energy-tests "No."]* "My father holds me back in life." *[He energy-tests "Yes."]* What does this mean to you?'

Man: 'It's a way of protecting myself.'

Vianna: 'Is your father stopping you from going to Australia?'

Man: 'If I look back, I can think of some links between him and my incapability to move back to Australia.'

Vianna: 'Repeat after me: "I'm scared about going back to Australia." *[He energy-tests "Yes."]* Why are you scared?'

Man: 'Maybe I'm afraid of getting stuck there.'

Vianna: 'So you think that once you go back, you'll have to stay there. Are you afraid of feeling disappointed by what you find there? Do you blame the Creator for this situation?'

Man: 'Well, I've often felt abandoned by the Creator and blamed God for things that happened to me.'

Vianna: 'Do I have permission to give you the programmes "I know how to trust in God" and "I know how to trust in my father" and the concept that you'll get home safely?'

Man: 'Yes.'

Vianna: 'Where's the pain now?'

Man: 'It's gone.'

DIGGING WORK EXAMPLE 15: LOVE

Vianna: 'Are you in love with somebody?'

Young woman: 'Yes, I am.'

Vianna: 'Is it the first time for you?'

Woman: 'It's the first time I have fallen in love this way.'

Vianna: 'How many times have you been in love?'

Woman: 'Three times.'

Vianna: 'What's different this time?'

Woman: '*I'm* different.'

Vianna: 'Tell me about this love you feel.'

Woman: 'I think he's the man I've always dreamed of.'

Vianna: 'So what's the matter?'

Woman: 'He's told me he loves me, but I'm scared. Maybe I won't be able to handle the relationship. I am afraid something terrible will happen.'

Vianna: 'What terrible thing could happen?'

Woman: 'He might leave me.'

Vianna: 'What would happen then?'

Woman: 'I'd feel angry and devastated.'

Vianna: 'And then?'

Woman: 'I'd ask him to come back.'

Vianna: 'And then?'

Woman: 'You'd think I would have learned something!'

Vianna: 'So what are you scared about?'

Woman: 'I'm afraid of letting myself go completely.'

Vianna: 'Repeat after me:

"I'm scared of letting myself go."

"I'm scared of loving."

"If I love too much, people leave me."'

The woman energy-tests 'Yes' to all.

Vianna: 'Has it always been like this?'

Woman: 'Yes, it has.'

Vianna: 'Would you like to live day to day without fearing anything?'

Woman: 'Yes, I would.'

Vianna: 'Repeat after me: "If they love me too much, I leave them." *[She energy-tests "Yes."]* Let's change this programme as well. Do I have your permission?'

Woman: 'Yes.'

Vianna: 'You fear love and the Creator's definition of being loved. What would happen if you stayed with this man and spent the next 30 years with him?'

Woman: 'I'd be happy.'

Vianna: 'What's wrong with this happiness?'

Woman: 'I'd be scared of being dumped. Maybe I wouldn't be able to satisfy him.'

Vianna: 'Why?'

Woman: 'I'm not good enough for him.'

Vianna: 'What do you mean? Have you ever had a long relationship with a man?'

Woman: 'Yes, I have.'

Vianna: 'What happened?'

Woman: 'It ended because we didn't love each other anymore.'

Vianna: 'Do you know how to maintain a long love story now?'

Woman: 'Yes, I think so.'

Vianna: 'Do you hate the man you left?'

Woman: 'No, but I felt irritated when I met him again. Now I'm OK.'

Vianna: 'Are you scared of leaving the man you love now, let's say in ten years?'

Woman: 'I'm scared of leaving him in a week as well as in ten years!'

Vianna: 'Why?'

Woman: 'I'm afraid I'm not enough for him and I won't be able to satisfy him.'

Vianna: 'Do you want to learn how to live feeling that you're enough? Have you ever felt that you're enough?'

Woman: 'Not really. It's been this way all my life.'

Vianna: 'Would you like to learn how to feel that you're enough and that you can express yourself freely? Let's teach you that you and this man are compatible and you can love each other.'

Woman: 'Yes!'

Vianna: 'How do you feel now?'

Woman: 'Very well!'

Vianna: 'Repeat after me:

"This relationship can contribute to my growth."

"I can love this man freely."

"I can accept his love freely."'

The woman energy-tests 'Yes' to all three.

Vianna: 'Sometimes our fear keeps love away from us. How do you feel now?'

Woman: 'I feel light.'

Vianna to class: 'She's still a bit scared of all the new feelings, but she'll get used to them.'

Vianna to woman: 'What do you think of your body?'

Woman: 'I find it hard to look at myself. I'm fat and I've got varicose veins, so I tend not to look at my legs. I love swimming and the seaside, but I can't stand the image of my body wearing a swimsuit. My sweetheart doesn't care if I'm ugly, but it matters to me.'

Vianna: 'What would happen if you accepted yourself as a whole?'

Woman: 'It would be too much.'

Vianna: 'For whom?'

Woman: 'For my parents. I was a danger to my father.'

Vianna: 'What does that mean?'

Woman: 'He was tough with me and I escaped from him more than once. And if I am too beautiful, my mother gets jealous. If I am too much of a woman, it is wrong.'

Vianna: 'Repeat after me:

"I'm scared of being too feminine."

"Being too much of a woman is wrong."

[She energy-tests "Yes" to both.]

131

"I'm safe if I'm a real woman."

[She energy-tests "No."]

'Would you like to live and be safe as a woman? To be beautiful and at the same time be safe from your father?'

Woman: 'Yes.'

Vianna: You escaped from him – what does that mean?'

Woman: 'Nothing. I loved him and I felt guilty for what I did.'

Vianna: 'What did you do?'

Woman: 'Nothing.'

Vianna: 'Would you like to live without feeling guilty? Do you love your husband as a father?'

Woman: 'Yes.'

Vianna: 'Repeat after me: "If I were beautiful I would leave my husband." *[She energy-tests "Yes."]* Would you like to have the chance to choose? Can I teach you that you can be beautiful and at the same time you can stay with your husband, because you love each other's souls?'

Woman: 'Yes.'

Vianna: 'Repeat after me: "I have to be the way I am now in order to stay with my husband. My husband is afraid that I would leave him if I were too beautiful." *[She energy-tests "Yes" to both.]* Do I have permission to download you with the feelings of "My legs are beautiful" and "My body is beautiful"?'

Woman: 'Yes.'

Vianna: 'How do you feel now?'

Woman: 'Better. But I'm not completely OK.'

Vianna: 'Do you like feeling beautiful? Your heart is afraid because I taught you new feelings.'

Woman: 'I don't know if I have the right to be beautiful. I've always judged beautiful people.'

Vianna: 'Do you think that beautiful people are stupid?'

Woman: 'Well, no – or maybe yes, they are! Or maybe they aren't stupid, but people are attracted by their appearance and nobody cares about their brain.

One can't be beautiful and at the same time be a good healer.'

Vianna: 'Does beauty frighten you? Are women afraid of beautiful women?'

Woman: 'I've been in competition with other women my whole life. I'm afraid I can't win if I express my intellect completely.'

Vianna: 'Repeat after me: "People take me seriously if I'm beautiful." *[She energy-tests "No."]* "If I'm beautiful, men won't come to me to be healed, but for other reasons." *[She energy-tests "Yes."]* Do I have permission to give you the programmes and feelings of "I can be respected by the men who are my clients and at the same time be beautiful" and "I know how to live without hiding"?'

Woman: 'OK.'

Vianna: 'I can see that you are stressed now. Why?'

Woman: 'Maybe it's about sex. My mother wanted me to be a nun.'

Vianna: 'Let's see... Repeat after me: "I am a nun." *[She energy-tests "Yes."]* "If I'm beautiful, it's wrong to have sex." *[She energy-tests "Yes."]* '

Woman: 'Sex makes me feel ill at ease, sort of strange.'

Vianna: 'Why does sex disturb you in that way?'

Woman: 'I'm afraid of being refused or considered stupid. I need to trust the other person completely to have sex.'

Vianna: 'Can I teach you how to feel good with sex?'

Woman: 'Yes.'

Vianna to class: 'She feels as if she has to choose between being a wife and a healer.'

Vianna to woman: 'Do I have permission to give you the feeling that you can be beautiful, both as a wife and as a healer?'

Woman: 'Yes.'

Vianna: 'How do you feel now?'

Woman: 'I feel wonderful. Much lighter! Thank you.'

Note to the reader: Because of being in a class environment, some issues were not addressed in this session. Can you sense what they are?

8

THE SEVEN PLANES OF EXISTENCE

The seven planes of existence are the seen and unseen forces of the cosmos. They are composed not only of the physical and 'known' universe but also the unseen forces that defy current scientific explanation. They are so vast that the human mind must be in an abstract state to comprehend them. The Theta state enables us to perceive these inexplicable forces in all their majesty through the Creator of All That Is. And in turn the planes of existence enable us to understand the glory of the Creator of All That Is.

As related in ThetaHealing, the concept of the seven planes of existence was introduced to me by the Law of Truth. It provides us with a vehicle for understanding how and why the world works on the physical and spiritual levels, and how this relates to us. The planes were set up for the development of humanity and naturally work together in a 'symphony' of cosmic order, though our belief systems can interfere with this. In some instances we can also become seduced by the 'brain candy' of the planes.

Each of the planes has its own particular energy, which is best described as a vibration, and is subject to its own conditions, rules, laws and commitments. Here is a brief summary of the characteristics of each of the planes. We will review them in more depth over the next few chapters.

The First Plane

The First Plane of Existence consists of all non-organic material on the Earth, all the elements that make up the Earth in its raw form and all the atoms of the periodic table before they start to bind to carbon bases. It is the minerals, the crystals, the soil and the rocks. It consists of every piece of Earth, from the smallest crystal to the largest mountain, in non-organic form.

The Second Plane

The Second Plane of Existence consists of organic material – vitamins, plants, trees, fairies and elementals. The molecular structure of this plane contains

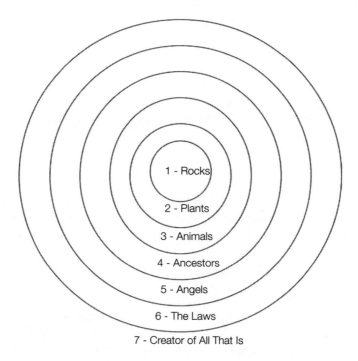

1 - Rocks

2 - Plants

3 - Animals

4 - Ancestors

5 - Angels

6 - The Laws

7 - Creator of All That Is

the first structures of a carbon molecule and is therefore organic matter. Minerals are non-organic and vitamins are organic; both are essential for life to occur.

The Third Plane

This is the plane where animals and humans exist. In part, we have created it for our own use. It is on this plane that we have the challenge of being governed by emotions, instinctual desires, passions and the reality of being in the human body in the physical world. This is the plane of protein-based life forms.

The Fourth Plane

The Fourth Plane of Existence is the realm of the spirit, where people live after death and where our ancestors are in waiting. This is what some people would consider the 'spirit world'.

The Fifth Plane

This is the plane of the ultimate in dualism. It is divided into hundreds of degrees. The lower degrees are where negative entities abide and the higher degrees are the realms of the angels, the Councils of Twelve that guide the soul families, the soul families themselves, the masters and our heavenly parents.

The Sixth Plane

This is the plane of the Laws, such as the Law of Time, the Law of Magnetism, the Law of Gravity, the Law of Light and many more Laws that create the very fabric of the universe.

The Seventh Plane

This is the plane of the Creator of All That Is. This is the level to use for instant healings and readings and the highest manifestations. It is a place of safety, love and 'It just is'.

CONNECTING TO THE PLANES

I believe that people who are intuitive begin to connect to the energies of the planes of existence as they develop their abilities. One of the benefits of the DNA activation is that it enables a person to connect with and walk through the planes of existence. Each strand of DNA in our body controls over 100,000 different functions. Therefore, it would be absurd to assume that the new DNA strands that are awakened with the DNA activation would only be associated with certain things, such as bliss, love and other emotions. Each new pair of chromosomes adds a new realm, a new understanding of the planes, giving new meaning to the phrase 'connected to All That Is'.

Each plane gives the seeker a vision of the divine filtered through it. I believe that this is how religions are formed. A connection is made with the consciousness of a plane and the belief systems of the plane are projected upon the seeker and go into the written word. We can become enamoured with the beauty and majesty of each plane, its belief systems, powers and healing properties.

We are influenced by all the planes of existence. We are part mineral, part of the plant kingdom because we consume it, part of the animal kingdom because we have a body, part of the spirit realm because we have a spirit. And because we live under the universal laws, we are connected to the Sixth Plane.

So, is it possible that you are sick because you are low on a mineral? Yes. But you may be low on a mineral because you're unable to absorb it because of an emotional programme. If you keep taking the mineral you're low on, will you work through the emotional programme? Eventually, yes. But we are connected to so many things, even to our ancestors – they are our connection to the DNA of the past – so, just when you think you're all together, you may be cleaning up programmes handed down to you genetically!

THE CONCEPT OF GOD

It has been suggested that many of us carry a genetic predisposition for belief in God, a 'God gene' if you will. This is not surprising, considering that it is likely that this predisposition would have survival benefits. These would likely be subtle, but in difficult times, what is more useful than belief in and communication with the Creator? In this communication, we connect to the divine essence that is within all of us and bring it into the physical world, thus enriching our lives.

Throughout history, humanity has been on a quest for God. Our perception of God is constantly changing and dependent on many influences, from the household to external society, religion and more recently modern science. The concepts of science are not necessarily *against* God, and were not designed as such. They were not a 'rebellion' against religion or God. Science is simple: it is an observation of our universe through explainable fact. The concept of God could be perceived as a science of its own – an observation of the universe that is spiritual and not always dependent upon physical causality but rather upon the unseen essence of thought and belief.

There are those who say that belief in God is an attempt to explain death and the hope of an afterlife. There does seem to be a pervading apprehension that once we die we will become nothing. One of the most prevalent fears that I see in people is 'fear of the nothing'. I believe that this belief stems from a superficial and materialistic view of the universe. I think that it is void of any imagination or self-love. My view is that we do not become nothing. You may ask, 'Then where do we go when we die?' I believe that once we have left the physical world, many of us transfer to a higher order of evolution. In this higher order, our abilities may be perceived as somewhat godlike by those still living on the Third Plane.

I believe that when we walk students up to the Seventh Plane we're taking them within their own brain to the message carriers, the neurons. They go within the very atomic energy that is in every atom. By doing this, their mind is stimulated with an awareness, an awareness that they are connected to every molecule, every atom and the energy associated with subatomic particles. This is the first step in ascension.

It will be this inner awareness that will bring us to the realization that we no longer have the need for the incredible competition of this world, and the battle of duality will be over. The massive power of the universe is within us, waiting for us to find it through focused thought. Once this power has been recognized within, it will flow outwards to the macrocosm of our everyday lives, expanding through the planes of existence to the immense macrocosm of the Seventh Plane of Existence and to the Creator of All That Is to become co-creation.

In the past, I believe that we have learned through experiencing one plane of existence at a time and learning its message. I believe that the message of the Fifth Plane is unconditional love. I believe that the message of the Sixth Plane is absolute truth and, perhaps, compassion. *I believe that now is the time that we are to become co-creators of our lives, consciously, awake and aware.*

PERCEIVING THE PLANES

Our perceptions of the planes is dependent upon our spiritual development or level of vibration. So the way that the energies of the first six planes is perceived is going to be different from person to person. For instance, two people are connecting to a particular angel from the Fifth Plane of Existence. These two people see the angel differently in their mind's eye. The reason why the essence of the same angel is seen differently by different people is that we are all vibrating at different frequencies. The essence of the angel is the same, but we are different. So there is no right or wrong in the perceptions of the two people, only different frequencies.

Understand that all the planes have their own particular frequencies and healing energies. The trick is knowing how to use the power inherent in each of them without being consumed by it. In order to gain mastership over the planes of existence, our *kundalini* must be awakened slowly, yet awakened nonetheless.

The deeper we get into a pure controlled Theta brainwave, the more it will become natural to access the planes through the Creator of All That Is of the Seventh Plane.

9

THE SEVENTH PLANE

The Seventh Plane is the pure energy of Creation; it is all-encompassing. This is the place of pure wisdom, of creative energy, of pure *love*, the place of instant healings, manifestations and the highest truth. It forms the other planes; it is the subatomic source of All That Is. It is the nucleus of the atom of creation. It holds the electrons, protons and neutrons that create life. These particles are the fountainhead of all life.

Through the Creator of All That Is of the Seventh Plane, instant healings, instant accountability and instant results are created. When healings are done from the Seventh Plane, we are under no obligation to honour the contracts and conditions that govern the first six planes of existence.

Each plane is divided by a thin *veil* that lies as a programme within the unconscious mind of every man, woman and child on this planet. When we go up to the Seventh Plane, we learn how to drop these veils so that we can realize that we are not *separate*, but connected to all of the planes. Once the mind (on a subconscious level) has made this leap (not by simply talking about it but by living it), the planes can be influenced to create manifestations and heal the physical body. This is the first time in the history of humanity that the planes of existence have been opened up simultaneously.

UNDERSTANDING THE SEVENTH PLANE

To reach an understanding of the Seventh Plane, you must first realize that the first six planes of existence are only illusions created by the inhabitants of each one. The pure truth is the Seventh Plane and the Creator of All That Is, the spirit that moves, intertwines and binds everything in existence. Some of my students refer to this energy as the 'Holy Spirit' and others refer to it as 'Source'. I refer to it as 'All That Is', the pure energy of the atom itself, the particles of protons. Regardless of what you call it, your pure intent, used with a Theta wave, is the deciding factor in accessing this energy of pure love.

With Seventh-Plane energy, you are consciously aware of every choice. You don't waste time on little idle things, such as drama, chaos and havoc. Issues are changed without self-criticism. Beliefs can be changed instantly. Once an understanding of this plane is reached, you attain the knowledge of Creation.

> *When using the Seventh Plane, you need to understand that this will increase your manifesting ability immediately. It is therefore important to avoid negative thoughts so that you do not manifest them.*

Vows, commitments and programmes can all block us from accessing the Seventh Plane and hence keep us from mastership of the planes.

Vows or Commitments to be Cleared in Order to Utilize the Seventh Plane

These are vows that most of us do not realize we have:

'I have to die to connect to God.'

'I have to suffer to be with God.'

'I have to die to prove my love of God or to please God.'

'I have to suffer to grow spiritually.'

'I have to die and return to grow spiritually.'

Programmes That Block Us from the Seventh Plane

These are as follows:

'I am afraid to own my power.'

Replace with: 'I understand what it feels like to have my own power' or 'I feel safe with my own power.'

'I have to be alone to get close to God.'

Replace with: 'I can be loyal to God and be with a companion' or 'I can love someone and be a healer.'

'I have to sacrifice one of my senses [such as the eyes and ears] to get close to God.'

Replace with: 'I am completely in tune with my body, mind and soul and have all my senses.'

HEALING FROM THE SEVENTH PLANE

When the healer connects to the Seventh Plane and witnesses the Creator's energy heal, the healing is done. It's that simple.

Healers working on this plane can achieve instant healings, though the client's free agency must be respected and their beliefs may be blocking the healing. However, on this plane, illness can simply be transformed into perfect health. And unlike the other planes, where the healer can be exhausted by the plane's vibration, this plane simply embraces the healer in love while it changes the human vibration to perfection.

Healers using this energy are themselves raised to perfect health. They can use all the planes without being bound by any oaths and commitments of the other planes. They will realize how to control their thoughts and experience instant manifestations that clear the limiting beliefs that bind them in fear.

Some healers are afraid of using this plane, thinking that they are going to God's God, but the Creator says you are just stepping into your birthright as a part of All That Is, without separateness.

10

THE SIXTH PLANE

The Sixth Plane of Existence has been called the great void. This plane is the Laws. There are Laws that govern our universe, our galaxy, our solar system, the Earth, and even us. There are Laws that govern all the other planes. It is because of these Laws that there is an imaginary division between the planes, though they truly exist altogether.

The Laws have a spirit-like essence, a living, moving consciousness. Throughout history there have been people who have been able to channel them to enable the vibration of humanity to ascend. Plato, Aristotle, Leonardo da Vinci, Galileo, Newton, Tesla, Edison and Einstein were all born with this ability. Tesla, for instance, channelled the Law of Magnetics and the Law of Electricity.

CALLING IN THE LAWS

In the days after I had first experienced the Laws in the form of huge faces in my living-room, my curiosity was piqued and I decided to experiment with them. When I had first talked to a Law, I had been scared because I hadn't known what it was. I'd thought I'd gone crazy. To prove to myself that it had been real, I decided to tell it to come back so that I could introduce it to my two friends. When it appeared in front of me and my friends, one of them fainted and the other saw bright spheres of light moving around the room.

My curiosity piqued even further; I decided to try an experiment with 17 people who had volunteered to help build an extra room for my office. We all settled into a discussion about psychic phenomena and the subject turned to the Laws. In spite of the fact that many of these people were *not* open-minded enough for this kind of thing, I decided to call the Laws in so they could experience them.

When I did, the Laws showed themselves as balls of light that floated around the room. When this happened, most of the people in the room fell asleep. Everyone who was still awake saw the lights, however, and one person wanted to talk to them. He wasn't very happy with all the spheres jumping around, but since he was a fan of cause and effect, he asked for the Law of Cause and Effect to come into this plane.

This Law came into my body with massive force. I felt an incredible weight, as though I was being slowly crushed. The Law began to use my body to speak to those in the group who were still awake. I felt detached from the process and just watched what was going on around me.

To test the Law, one person asked it, 'What is emotion?' The Law then started to choke me to show them it knew what emotion was. I was turning blue when Mark, one of my good friends, came to my rescue. He commanded that the Law leave my body. It did leave and I started to breathe again in deep gasps.

Having that Law in my space nearly killed me. That's how I realized it was permissible to send your consciousness to the Sixth Plane and talk to the Laws to learn knowledge, but to 'call in' the Laws, one or many, to this plane was *not* a good idea. These energies are what move the universe. They are incredibly powerful and it is difficult for the human body to utilize the full force of a Law within it. So do not ever permit these energies into your space. You should always speak to these beings through the Seventh Plane of Existence.

HEALING FROM THE SIXTH PLANE

Anytime tones, colours, numbers, magnetism, sacred geometry, the Earth's magnetic grid, astrology and numerology are used in healings, a healer is tapping into the Laws of the Sixth Plane of Existence. Here there is the knowledge of tones that balance the body perfectly and change the vibration of any virus. The philosophy on the Sixth Plane is 'If it's broken, fix it.'

Healers using the Sixth Plane of Existence realize that they are living in an illusion and that they are directing their own illusion. They know they no longer need to punish themselves in order to progress. On this plane, the battle between good and evil is eliminated and replaced by pure truth.

One of the Laws that you will tap into when doing Theta work is the Law of Truth, which will help you all through your life.

To activate a Law, you must first go to the Seventh Plane. If you want to anchor the energy of the Law in order to apply that energy, you must first ask for the name of the Law. The name is a tone or vibration that will activate the Law. Then you wait for the energy, vibration and information to come to you.

It is also on the Sixth Plane that we learn to access the Hall of Records, where information about people's life experiences is held, by holding a proper Theta Delta state to create a vision of ourselves accessing the hall.

VORTICES OF THE SIXTH PLANE

Many years ago, when I was first dating Guy, I would drive out to Roberts, Idaho, to visit him. The Roberts area has its own peculiar weather patterns, especially in winter. As the sun warms the air, moisture rises up from the Snake river, causing a mist to form that is sometimes so thick it is difficult to drive safely. When the temperature drops suddenly, the mist will flow through the areas close to the river. For a psychic, this mist is a portal that makes it easy to see all kinds of psychic phenomena.

The whole area can be an eerie place and this was particularly true of where Guy was living at that time. The road to his house was named Stibal Lane, after his great grandfather, who had first settled there. Legend had it that at the entrance to Stibal Lane from the larger road of Bassett there was a Native American burial ground. People in the area had seen spectres of Native Americans dressed in ancient clothing walking along that part of Stibal Lane. There had been other strange sightings, too, particularly when the mist formed from the winding Snake river. One night Guy and I saw a curious sight ourselves.

Guy tells the story:

In the winter of 1997 Vianna and I had just met and were dating one another. We were living in separate homes and would visit each other whenever we could. I was working on the ranch and Vianna was doing readings, so we were both very busy. We would take turns visiting each other and on one of those misty winter nights peculiar to the Roberts area, it was Vianna's turn to come out to see me.

Late that night she had to leave to get home to her daughter Bobbi, who was pregnant at the time. We were in the throes of new love and, wanting to spend as much time with her as I could, I walked her out to her car. Night had fallen and with it a blanket of thick mist had formed. As we walked out to where she had parked her car, we saw two columns of slow, swirling energy about 30 feet high. They looked like slow-moving pearlescent white dust devils. One of them was close to Vianna's car and, laughing, she walked into the middle of it and imitated its swirling movement with her arms. Stepping out of it, she explained to me that these were vortices – portals openings between dimensions. I was curious about them, but

Vianna had no time to explain further. She jumped into her car and took the slow drive through the mists towards Idaho Falls.

She called me when she got home and began to tell me what she knew about vortices. A vortex is a positive and negative ionized energy field that creates an opening between dimensions, space and time. There are many different types of vortices. Some are natural and others are created through thought forms or sometimes even rituals.

A vortex gives you the opportunity to create great change, but its energy can benefit you only if you are in a good space. So, before you experience one, make sure you are centered in yourself. If you are not, the vortex will pull your energy in different directions. You can wear an amulet that is a chakra balancer and protector, such as charoite or labradorite, to help keep you centered on your life's plan and mission.

Vortices are around us more than we realize, and all of us, to a greater or lesser extent, are vortices in and of ourselves.

The body's nervous system can sense and even create vortex energy. This may bring out the good or the bad in others. A healer should be a controlled vortex to bring out whatever needs to be cleared in a person, but this can be challenging when their very presence brings up someone's issues. When a person has overwhelmingly negative belief systems, it is important that their space is entered through the Creator of All That Is of the Seventh Plane of Existence. If an intuitive enters their space using the third eye, they will trigger their programmes. The intuitive will then begin to react to these programmes, assuming that the client and the practitioner have these programmes in common, and may begin acting them out in the way that they treat the person. For example, the client may have the programme that no one cares and they are not important. Unless the practitioner is in tune with the process, they may become busy and the client may feel ignored. It is important not to react to this vortex energy that a person creates from negative programmes.

To see vortex energy created by programmes, command to 'see' a person's space directly from your third eye and watch the energy as it swirls and pulses around the person. This is done in a similar way to seeing someone's aura.

Uncontrolled vortex energy in a person can influence their own behaviour as well as that of the people around them. In an intuitive person, electrical pulses of the body (which are vortex energy) cause an iridescent ultraviolet light to be released from the body's nervous system, affecting the mind-body-soul in various ways. This is manifested outward in different ways. Bees will be drawn to you, electrical appliances will be affected and spirits may appear to you. To deal with these challenges, command that your energy be balanced and that all wayward spirits that come around you be sent to God's light.

11

THE FIFTH PLANE

When my business began to take off in 1998, I worked long hours. I would sometimes become a little melancholy at being cooped up in my office doing readings all day. One day, during a rare break, I wistfully looked out the window and thought of all the things that I would like to do and of the faraway places that I would like to see. I had an hour's lunch break between readings, so I decided to go to those places another way – to escape for a little while through meditation.

I asked my friend Chrissie to do a crystal layout for me. A crystal layout is a guided imagery technique that is designed to help a person envisage going to other places and times with the eye of the mind. I lay down on the massage table that we used for the journeys, and Chrissie set up the crystals in a grid around my body. She placed her hands on my head, and her calm and rhythmic voice guided me into the cosmos, past space and time.

All of a sudden I was in the middle of a full-blown vision. As clearly as if I was standing there in the flesh, I found myself in what I can only describe as a courtroom furnished in dark polished wood. Arranged around the courtroom were magnificent men and women who seemed to emanate light. One of them stepped forward and said to me, 'You're late. Come in and take your place at the front!'

'Oh,' I said, 'I'm sorry, I was in my body on Earth. I had no idea it was time for court.'

I was astonished at myself for saying this and yet this whole scenario was suddenly eerily familiar to me. I knew that I had been here before and I had seen all these beings in another time. What made it more bizarre was that I knew in a flash why I was in this place now.

One of the beings escorted me to the centre of the court to the place of the defence lawyer. To the right of me stood a tall man in a grey cloak with long white hair. His eyes twinkled with glee as he met my gaze. I knew that this was the god Odin, my old adversary. He smiled, and when he spoke to me, his voice was beautiful to hear. It reached into me as music does when one hears a heartfelt song for the first time.

'So,' he said, 'once again I see you have come to be the advocate for humanity! For a while there I thought you weren't going to show up. Will you always attempt to save them?'

I didn't fall into the trap set by his magic voice and shrugged off the lilting tones that he sent at me.

'Your magic tricks won't work on me, Odin. You know I will fight for them as I always have!'

The banter between us was good-natured, because, you see, Odin and I were not enemies – at least not in the general sense. Let us say that we had a difference of opinion pertaining to the human race... You see, these beings were caretakers of the human race. At this time and place, it was up to them to decide if it should be permitted to continue or destroyed as a civilization and its souls reassigned to other places. Some in the courtroom were in favour of destruction and renewal, while others were like me – advocates for the continuance, nurturing and teaching of humans.

The judge banged his gavel down and said, 'Court is in session! We will hear arguments from the esteemed god Odin [*Odin inclined his head at the compliment*], who is the advocate for the destruction of the human race as it now is and for it to be rebuilt from the very beginning, with the last remaining seeds of humanity spread through the stars to begin anew to be cleansed of all wickedness, vice and evil. The advocate for humanity is, as always, the venerated representative of the Goddess, who will argue against the destruction of all humanity.'

I inclined my head and said, 'It is once again a pleasure, your honour.'

'We first will hear the argument for the destruction of all humanity from the god Odin. Proceed.'

Odin smiled and began to speak, his voice seductive and filled with persuasiveness. He spread his hands, indicating the audience.

'Your honour, esteemed ascended masters and angels of the most high! We are gathered here once again to judge the merits of the human race. I find its destruction to be the only recourse that we can follow. I need only to direct your attention to history up until the present time.'

A vortex opened in the centre of the courtroom and the history of humanity began to unfold in a three-dimensional hologram.

'Look at them! From the dawn of agriculture, we have seen the beginnings of war. The lust for wealth, power and resources has been insatiable. We have seen how they have in a short 10,000-year period repeatedly stripped to the bone the very land that does its best to feed them. Look how they have created the entity of war upon one another for the sake of greed and self-glory. They have wantonly destroyed whole ecosystems and thousands of species with them! They have enslaved other species for food and for beasts of burden. Why, they have even enslaved one another! Look, my fellow celestials, how they have permitted a few among them to be kings and queens because they were too lazy to rule themselves. Look at how these early peoples fell from the innocence that once was and created the age of metals to master fire. This was when things really went off-kilter. As their power grew and technology took hold, its clawed hand began to poison the minds of men and women in a lust to dominate their surroundings and subjugate every living thing on the Earth to the will of humankind.

'Harken! This is not the worst that has been done, for there are sins that are more subtle. Each one of you knows that part of our mission as celestials is to bring sacred knowledge to humanity from time to time, bringing men and women divine inspiration in the way of philosophy and religion, with rituals and symbolism that enrich and stimulate the hearts of these pitiful creatures. Each of you knows how you have been rewarded for your troubles. Name me one philosophy, one religion, one magical tradition, that has been left in the purity in which it was given! Name me one!'

Odin's blazing eyes and magical voice went out into the audience like a shock wave.

'In all the time that I have been an emissary of this court I have never seen one instance in all the annals of human history where sacred knowledge has not been twisted, added to, changed, altered and misused to the point that any resemblance of the original divinity was utterly destroyed. I challenge even one of you to give me one instance where purity and innocence have not been lost! Oh, and lest we forget the last 4,000 years of mounting warfare and the wholesale slaughter of innocent people on both sides of warring factions…! I must admit, to me war once served a purpose – that of whittling down the numbers of this dangerous and violent species. But, as we can see, even war cannot keep up with the billions that are on the planet now. Need I mention the crimes of murder, incest, rape, child abuse, substance abuse and corruption? Need I mention starving people and genocide? Does the court really want me to go on? I believe that I have made my point and clearly stated my case for the destruction and reseeding of humanity, to begin anew, fresh and unsullied by the evil that so persists in the hearts of all humans.'

With that, Odin turned to me, beamed a warm smile at me and said, 'Your turn.'

The hologram blinked out of existence.

The judge said: 'We will now hear arguments from the representative of the mother Goddess.'

From inside me I could feel the power building. I raised my arms above my head as though I was holding something. A pulsing light began to shine from my hands. The light began to build until all those in the room were blinded by the brilliance of what I held in my hands. In a flash, I was holding a beautiful tiny baby. There was a pearly luminescence coming from it and I could hear myself speaking with a strong voice that reverberated throughout the courtroom. 'What about *this*?' I said as I indicated the shining baby for all to see, turning in a circular motion and meeting the eyes of each in the assembly. 'I hold in my hands the essence of innocence!'

The little baby began to laugh with a sound like the tinkling of tiny silver bells. The laughter permeated the room with an essence of purity, touching the heart of each being in the courtroom.

'Look,' I said to the assembly, 'so perfect and pure! I believe that each of us should defend humanity with every prayer!'

For long moments there was utter silence in the courtroom until the judge brought his gavel smashing down. 'Case dismissed!' he said. 'Humanity will continue as it has been. You still have your timeline. Proceed as planned.'

At that moment I came to the realization that for a brief instant in time I was one of many defence lawyers for humankind and I was the representative of all the millions of positive wishes to save the world. I believe that it is the inner wish of all healers to uphold this responsibility.

Then I was taken from the courtroom into the past, to the time when it all began, the time when we of the Fifth Plane of Existence agreed to the responsibility of watching over our children, the human race…

CHILDREN OF THE MASTERS

To explain who we are, why we are on this planet and how we relate to the planes of existence, we will start with this simple outline.

Our spirits begin as essences of energy in the Fifth Plane as children of the masters. A master of the Fifth Plane is an enlightened being who has learned to manipulate time, matter and subatomic particles. When we are born as children on the Fifth Plane, we have great creative abilities. But, like all children, we must learn proper discernment in using these abilities. So, as children of pure energy, we are sent on an immense journey beyond space and time, leaving the Fifth Plane to go to the Fourth Plane of Existence, the spirit world. Here we are tutored, nurtured and loved, and are given different assignments, according to our abilities.

First we are sent to the First Plane to understand it completely, to learn the molecular structure of the mineral kingdom and the building blocks of inorganic matter. Once this knowledge as been assimilated, we return to the Fourth Plane to report. Everything that we have learned is recorded. Then we are sent to the Second Plane, to the realm of the plants, to study them. Then we return to the Fourth Plane to report these experiences. In fact, it may be these young spirits that some perceive as fairies.

Once we have mastered these two planes, we are sent to the Third Plane, where we learn about the flesh and blood physical body. In the mortal body, we learn to make decisions and create from the challenges of the physical.

From the physical plane, we learn to overcome the physical body and control our thoughts, and are allowed the opportunity to come to the realization that we are made up of All That Is. We learn to create with All That Is through our mind, projecting thoughts from the physical and reclaiming our status as co-creators. There is an old saying: 'I think, therefore I am.' My saying would be 'I think, therefore I am part All That Is' or 'I am, therefore I think.'

The Third Plane of Existence is also the place to overcome dysfunctional programmes. This is one reason why we come here.

One of the best reasons to release these programmes is because they can be manifested into existence. For instance, if I truly believe something, then I'll draw it right to me. This is because the subconscious is run by the most prevalent thought within it. The signal of this thought is projected outward and the world treats us accordingly. So, for instance, a person might bring into this incarnation the belief of 'I'm strong – I'll take your punishment' and then take punishment for others all their life.

What is sad is that we may be so comfortable with a belief that we may not know that we have it or that it is dysfunctional. Some of the most self-destructive beliefs are carried with us like a wolf in sheep's clothing, hiding in plain sight.

The cycle of learning continues until the Third Plane is mastered and we are given the chance to return to the Fifth Plane. Everyone that has ascended to the Fifth Plane can do amazing things because they have learned that their spiritual essence is not separate from the Creator. They have learned how to rejuvenate the physical, mental, emotional and spiritual bodies.

When we have completed this learning process, we can take our place with our spiritual parents as masters on the Fifth Plane to create with control and proper discernment. The parents themselves are still evolving, learning to use and master the Seventh Plane, until they reach the highest level of progress and become part of the Sixth Plane.

The Third Plane of Existence was actually created so the parents could watch their children progress. Until recent times they were permitted to do no more than this. Now they are permitted to participate. What is happening now is that ascended masters are coming to the Third Plane on a mission to help their children save humanity.

In this instance, the ascended master comes to Earth and is born as a child. A child in the womb by its very nature has immeasurable innocence and purity, because it is so close to the Creator. It is only through this purity that it is possible for a master to inhabit the flesh for long periods of time. In an act of self-surrender, the master condenses their vast energies and lowers their vibration to inhabit the embryo. As the child grows into a adult, the master slowly rises to the high frequency of their true nature. This is one of the ways in which a marriage is made between the Third and Fifth Planes.

Some Fifth-Plane beings have such magnificent energy that they require more than one human body to encompass them and inhabit more than one person at a time.

There can be drawbacks to inhabiting a human body, however, in that once a master becomes a newborn child, the memories of who they were in the prior incarnation are sometimes suppressed. The majority of the masters who have come on a mission to this plane do not immediately remember who they are. As they grow up, they sense that there is so much more to themselves, but struggle to remember what it is. In time, they remember who and what they are. I refer to them as Rainbow Children.

At some point in time, they do remember their mission:

1. They must relearn how to use the Seventh Plane and clear their limitations and then teach this process.

2. They must teach their students how to have discipline in their thoughts and how to tap into All That Is.

Once a master's memory begins to return, the first realization that they have is that they don't belong here. They have strange feelings like 'I'm in the wrong family, and someday the right family will find me' or 'I am on the wrong planet.' It is their soul family that they are yearning for and they begin to look for incarnations of these spiritual beings in human form in the people they meet. In many instances they will meet a person and recognize them as being one of the members of this family who is here on a mission as well. The recognition of these soul family members will be strong and the memories will return to remind them that that they were once in a spiritual family of a high frequency.

In some instances these feelings and memories will bring two people together in matrimony. But this is like a brother and a sister marrying without knowing it. There is a difference between a soul family member and a soul mate. Soul families are drawn together to do the work of the Creator. They descend to inhabit physical families on this plane. Soul mates, on the other hand, have been in passionate love that spans time and many planes of existence.

ThetaHealing is collecting soul families together to do the work of the Creator. It is designed to bring them together again.

The same scenario of the planes that is being played out in this world is happening all across the galaxies in other civilizations as a means of teaching the branches of our soul families in those places.

As we on the Third Plane become more aware of ourselves and our surroundings, the illusion of the Third Plane will disappear. This does not mean that we are creating the world as a hologram for us to play in and it is only us in the hologram. On a soul level, we are all cognizant of this illusion and are all living in it together, though separated by our belief systems. One of the major lessons we are here to learn is to have respect for ourselves and for one another.

HEALING FROM THE FIFTH PLANE

People who channel angels and prophets and bring spirits in to perform psychic surgery are tapping into this plane of existence. Healers using this energy are bound by the 'rules' of the Fifth Plane and will often heal with a sacrifice of energy.

On the lower levels of this plane, *ego* still resides. Negative programmes such as 'I must be punished', 'It's selfish to heal myself' and 'I must battle evil all the time' should be cleared to use this plane. (More programmes are given in *ThetaHealing*.) If you have the programme of 'I have to battle evil', for instance, it is possible that you will draw evil energies in order to battle with them. This programme should be replaced with 'I am impervious to evil'. This is not to say that there is no evil in the world, just that if you have this programme you will not draw it to you. Other programmes to instill are:

'I am always safe.'

'I know what it feels like to be safe.'

'I know how to live without anger.'

'I know how to live with faith.'

'I know the Creator's definition of what faith feels like.'

'I know how to live without fear.'

Make sure that there are no commitments that you have to be alone to be a healer, or that you have to trade one of your senses to gain power, or that you have any vows or commitments from another place or time (see

ThetaHealing for a full list). Some people have the beliefs that you are not allowed to defend yourself or protect yourself, or that you have to permit people to control you. These should be pulled and replaced.

As explained in *ThetaHealing*, when healers attempt to tap into the Fifth Plane, they first tap into the boundaries of the Third Plane, for example with the programmes 'I am mortal' or 'I have limits'. It's important to remember that these boundaries were only put in place in order for us to move above them and go back to the Fifth Plane.

Also remember that if you're working with a Fifth-Plane consciousness, your ego may interfere with your judgement. You'll refuse to look at the possibility of not being right or to work on yourself. Be alert for this.

Spirits of the Fifth Plane can act as mediators between humans and the Creator of All That Is, but also be alert for the fact that these beings inadvertently interject their own opinions into the information and this can be confusing. One should learn from this plane, not get swept up in the drama of the battle of good against evil or get bogged down by the opinions of the beings of this plane.

Each plane has its own version of truth, but the Seventh Plane is the highest truth. So when you receive information from a Fifth-Plane spirit, go up and verify the information with the Creator of All That Is. On the Seventh Plane, all information is available to those who ask and the Creator will always help you.

PSYCHIC ATTACK, NEGATIVE INFLUENCES

Have you ever felt that you have been hit by a psychic attack? What if you were impervious to these influences? Spirits, negative thought forms, evil energy – what if these things were gone from your life?

People who do a lot of healing and psychic work can be affected by these influences. Both healer and client can get tied up in a particular plane of existence and use only that plane's energy in the healing. One of the planes that healers use extensively is the Fifth Plane and this is the plane of battle, of good against evil in a constant conflict. This conflict is connected to and played out in the Third Plane. But what if there were no need for this conflict and you could tap into a plane that just was? What if you could tap into total unconditional love and be protected, strong, healthy and at the centre of all things? What if another person's anger did not affect you because you could intuitively see where they were coming from and could diffuse their anger with this understanding? Is this where you want to be? These energies are on the Seventh Plane of Existence.

PROTECTION AND GUIDANCE FROM ANGELS

As an exercise in how to use the Fifth Plane of Existence energy, you can send an angel to protect and guide another person. If directed from the Seventh Plane, the angel will simply protect the person and not become involved in the drama of good and evil.

THE PROCESS TO DIRECT A GUARDIAN ANGEL

1. Centre yourself in your heart and visualize yourself going down into Mother Earth, which is a part of All That Is.

2. Visualize bringing up energy through your feet, opening up all of your chakras as you go. Go up out of your crown chakra, in a beautiful ball of light, to the universe.

3. Go beyond the universe, past the white lights, past the dark light, past the white light, past the jelly-like substance that is the Laws, into a pearly iridescent white light, into the Seventh Plane of Existence.

4. Gather unconditional love and make the command to the Creator of All That Is: *'Creator, it is commanded that a guardian angel protect this person. Thank you. It is done. It is done. It is done.'*

5. Witness the guardian angel going into the person's space to protect them.

6. Imagine being rinsed off. Imagine your energy coming back into your space and going down into the Earth. Pull the Earth energy up through all your chakras to your crown chakra.

7. Make an energy break.

12

THE FOURTH PLANE

When I began to do readings professionally for the first time, I began to have visionary dreams, both asleep and awake, with increased intensity. In retrospect, I believe that these were dreams of initiation into the planes of existence. Each vision was leading me to explore the planes; each was a guide to perceiving the nuances associated with a particular plane. Some of them happened when I was close to water. I believe the reason for this is that water is a good conductor of electrical energy. A visionary portal often seems to be made when I am sitting in a warm tub of water, relaxing after a long day of readings.

One of the most intense and harrowing of these early visionary experiences taught me one of my most important lessons. The first part came in a dream when I was sleeping.

I found myself in what looked like the desert mountains of Arizona. It was night-time and I was sitting close to a camp fire that was burning brightly in the darkness. The vision was so real that I could feel the heat of the fire on my skin as the wind fanned the flames.

Across from me sat a Native American man. The power that emulated from him set my teeth on edge. He looked very strange. His hair was twisted and matted with feathers sticking out in all directions and seemed to be tied up in a partial bun of some sort. His face was painted black on one side and white on the other. He sat staring at me motionless for some time, then all of a sudden got up and began to sing and dance around the fire. As he danced, he began to make strange animal-like noises. I sat transfixed, frozen in place, unable to move as I watched the primaeval dance.

Then he began to speak in some kind of old Native American tongue. I do not know how, but somehow I could understand him.

He said, 'Today, if you want the power of the *shapeshifter*, I can give it to you. But you must abide by certain rules.'

Without waiting for my reply, he picked up a wicked-looking obsidian axe from his side and came at me with it. As fast as thought, he swung the axe in a glittering arc over his head. I wasn't quick enough to evade his lightning movement and the axe struck me as I was rising to stand up. I felt it biting deep into me. It sliced me open from the top to the bottom of my chest, opening my sternum. Out of this open wound in my body I transformed into a beautiful golden eagle, as though I was bursting forth from an egg.

Now in the form of the eagle, I spread my wings in an effort to escape. But before I could rise into the air, the Native American screamed at me: 'Look!' He slashed with the axe at the breast of the eagle. Out of this open wound came a mountain lion.

In the form of the mountain lion, I slashed about myself with my claws and snarled at the man. He screamed at me again: 'Look!' With uncanny speed he slashed at me again. Unable to escape, I could only watch helplessly as he slashed open the breast of the mountain lion I had become. Out of this wound came a screaming falcon that flew into the air.

Still there was no escape. Once again the man screamed at me: 'Look!' and sliced open the shape I had become. Out of the open wound came a great black, brown and grey female timber-wolf.

Finally, this felt right. The wolf was me; I was the wolf. I felt a strange sense of familiarity, as though I had become the wolf many times before. I felt the freedom and passion that only comes from being a wild animal. In a rush, I remembered all the times I had run with the wolves in my dreams and in all the lives that I had experienced before. Suddenly I remembered my excruciating experiences when I had had cancer in this life. When I think of that time, it is the intense pain that returns to me, like the ancient genetic memory of the teeth of a carnivore tearing into my flesh. The pain often became so intense that I would astral travel to leave my body and run with a wolf pack in the Montana mountains. At first, I ran with them in human form, but after a while I would jump inside the wolves and become part of the pack. And as I ran with this wolf pack, I would search for my man from Montana.

This all came back to me in a flash as I stood on four legs in front of the Native American in the form of a mighty female timber-wolf, staring at him intently through green eyes that were still human.

He said to me, 'These are the rules of the shapeshifter: you must not cut your hair for six years. Three years from now I will come to you again to give you guidance. In six years you will learn to master the power of the shapeshifter. You must follow my instructions or you will be lost.'

When I woke from the dream, my sternum was sore to the touch. Two or three days afterwards, Guy and I were in a terrible car wreck. I was thrown forward with such violence that the seatbelt broke my sternum.

When I was healed, the dream began to haunt me. There seemed to be a correlation between it and the wreck, but I didn't know what it was. I did know that I was going through a 'little death', a initiation process to become a shapeshifter that might end up with me getting killed in order to wield the power. So the first thing I did was to cut my hair because that was the thing the man had told me I shouldn't do.

I think when I cut my hair it was an act of pure defiance.

I had begun to notice that many intuitive people only focused on one particular plane of existence at a time, and the rules attached to it, and had started to realize, through these visionary experiences, that there had to be a single all-encompassing energy of *All That Is*, an energy that you could tap into to make things happen without having to follow specific rules from different dimensions and incarnations. I'd had the enlightenment of the All That Is of the Seventh Plane of Existence explained to me by the Laws of the Sixth Plane, so I began to question the rules attached to the different energies of the planes and how I could transcend them.

Six years to the day from the first dream, I was relaxing in the bathtub after a long day of work. I closed my eyes for a moment and suddenly I was once again within a vision in that mountain place in Arizona. The flames from the same fire rose into the sky and licked the darkness. There he was, the magnificent Native American, on the other side of the fire, staring at me through the flames with his painted face and strange hair.

He spoke to me in that same old dialect that I could somehow understand: 'You have earned the right to become a shapeshifter. I will teach you the secrets of shapeshifting and you will remember them from before.'

It was at this moment that I remember staring at him long and hard and saying, '*No, thank you.* I do not choose to follow you or to learn from you. I only choose to follow the Creator of All That Is.'

He seemed annoyed and said, 'But look! I can give you this power to use as you so choose. This is a great and wonderful power! Take it, it is yours!'

'Truly, this thing that you offer is great,' I told him. 'But the true and wonderful power is the Creator of All That Is. I do not need to take this gift that you offer. It is the *Creator* who is the master of this gift. Through the Creator, I can create it myself. Thank you, but please leave.'

The man bowed his head in what seemed to be resignation. A hush seemed to fall over the vision; even the crackling of the fire became quiet. A vast stillness seemed to grow all about me. Out of this stillness I heard a voice speak from every direction at once. It said: '*You have passed the test. Your initiation is complete. You have done well, my child.*'

The Native American looked at me with those fierce, soulful eyes of his and said, 'That was the right answer. Congratulations.'

I came back to myself in the bathwater with the realization that something important had happened to me, but what came next was truly profound.

As I lay in the warm water, a divine presence came to me and I was directed to send my consciousness up to the place where I had always gone before. I did as I was directed and sent my consciousness to 'Go Up and Seek God'. (I didn't know it at the time, but this was to my heavenly father on the Fifth Plane of Existence.) As I bathed in this divine presence, the incredible essence of my heavenly father spoke to me and said: 'It is time. Come with me to the Seventh Plane.'

I was confused. I thought that this *was* the Seventh Plane and that this *was* the Creator. After all, it was so divine, so serene and beautiful here. I had done so many healings from this place. How could there possibly be anywhere beyond it?

Sensing my confusion, my heavenly father explained, 'Up until this time you have only plugged into the Seventh Plane of Existence to do your healings. Come, and we will take you to that plane so that you can be present there and truly experience it without being separate from it.'

I was confused by all this. I had gone to the Laws for many answers and I was terrified of going to a place that was beyond them. I was afraid that I would turn into pure light or energy and would be released from my body. I was terrified that Guy would walk in and find nothing left but my clothes and a bathtub full of water.

I spoke of my fear to my heavenly father. He began to comfort me, telling me that everything would be fine. Yes, he told me, I would change, but I would not become pure light because I was already a part of God, a part of creation.

Trusting in my heavenly father, I decided to take the next step forward. I imagined myself going up past the Laws. I passed through a membrane of jelly-like substance and imagined myself going up until I was in the very place of creation, the creative energy of All That Is.

In that moment I realized that I had never been separate from God. I realized that what my human mind-body had perceived as an illusion was part of the energy of All That Is. I realized we are *all* a part of All That Is. There is *no separation*.

From that time onward the healings became more effective. And yet at the same time something strange happened inside me: I no longer felt that I had to *fix* everyone. I could watch people live their lives and go through their learning processes with detachment. Before that time I had tried to correct people's problems using whatever plane they were learning from. I would attempt to get them focused on going to the place that I thought was right. I now realized that the Creator energy of All That Is was all around us and I found a way to drop the veil of separation. I found a way to look at humans with a different perspective, through simple observance.

I don't own any books that tell me about the energy of All That Is. Philosophy is a nice thing, but can become over-idealistic and lost in ideas. The message that I received moved an idealistic idea into a reality, one that you can use in the physical world *at will*. This was the beginning of DNA 3. DNA 3 is the ability to *create at will*.

When I passed the Fourth-Plane initiation with the Native American, it was the last barrier for me. This initiation opened up a new level of consciousness.

The planes of existence are numbered from one to seven. But the initiations of these planes can happen at any time on any plane, depending on your spiritual development and vibration. The only reason that the planes are numbered is to give the mind enough brain candy to understand them. I went through the planes of existence initiations in a roundabout fashion myself. I was initiated into the First Plane of Existence first. Then I was initiated into the Fifth Plane, then the Sixth, then the Second and lastly the Fourth, to be led to where I am today.

An initiation into the planes does not have to be a death door initiation or involve the stipulation that you have to die to progress. The trick is to go through the Seventh Plane *first* to find out what the initiations are and experience them through the Creator of All That Is. The lesson of the Fourth Plane of Existence for me was not to get caught up in the brain candy and to stay focused on the essence of the Seventh Plane of the Creator of All That Is.

From that day forward I began teaching the planes of existence with more intensity than ever before. On that day I was given a way to focus the mind to get to the right place to ask questions and to create healings; to go to the place where there is no opinion, only truth. It was through this initiation that I was able to find the road map to the Creator of All That Is.

It was after this that my perceptions of the fundamental nature of God began to change radically. For instance, take the word 'God'. Think about the belief systems around that word. For many, it seems to generate issues concerning humanity's worthiness to connect to God. I found that some people had difficulty going up to the Seventh Plane of Existence of the Creator of All That Is using the singular term 'God', mainly because of their perceptions of the word. To answer this challenge, the command process was permanently changed to *'Father, Mother, God, Creator of All That Is, it is commanded…'*

As the teachings progressed and ThetaHealing touched more people, I saw that some people would consistently connect to the Creator of All That Is and others would get lost along the way. I knew that I had to find a way for everyone to connect to the highest plane without interference from their ego and the beliefs that bound them. In response to this need I began to explain the planes of existence in more depth. A conceptual path to the Creator of All That Is for everyone was forming.

THE REALM OF SPIRIT

The Fourth Plane is the plane where we learn to master the spirit, or what we perceive as the spiritual aspect of Creation. It is the place between life and death and the doorway to the realms beyond death. When we die, our carbon-based body is laid to rest, but our ATP goes forward to the Fourth Plane of Existence. From there, some spirits will choose to stay as spirits, others will choose to incarnate again and yet others will move to other planes.

As a spirit, we still have essence, and can still feel, hear, taste and touch. Surely these feelings are not experienced in the same sense on the Fourth Plane as on the Third, but it is similar. There we can feel the air run right through us and can feel the essence of fresh-baked bread. Our senses are actually better than on the Third Plane. New colours become apparent to us and new things can be heard.

On the Fourth Plane we still eat and still have to give ourselves nutrition. This world is simply one of a higher vibration, where the molecules are moving faster than on the Third Plane. No plane is really 'solid' – they are all simply different combinations of energy, vibration and light.

Many highly evolved guides come from the Fourth Plane. This is where the children of the Fifth Plane first learn about creation.

HEALING FROM THE FOURTH PLANE

This plane offers access to the *spiritual ancestors*. Shamans and medicine men often use their ancestors and other spirits to aid them in healing, using both the ancestors' wisdom itself and the healing or herbs suggested by them. In this way they make an 'equation' between the Second, Third and Fourth Planes of Existence (an equation is using more than one plane of existence at a time).

Healers that understand the specific healing energy of this plane are, however, restricted by the obligations of consciousness that exist here. To recap briefly:

- People using this plane for healing believe that the healer cannot heal themselves. This is the plane of exchanging one thing for another, of taking a person's sickness upon yourself and then getting rid of it.

- Healers connected to Fourth Plane energies have a programme that it is wrong to accept money for healing sessions; only gifts are accepted.

- This plane, like other planes, teaches via initiations. There are beliefs on this plane that say a person has to come close to death or even die to learn more – to master the plane, they must dance with death or die the 'little death' of initiation.

- The initiation of this plane is self-sacrifice. The idea is that we must suffer to learn, to overcome the beliefs of our ancestors and to overcome the material world and the beliefs surrounding it.

- Spirits on the Fourth (and Fifth) Plane of Existence can be misleading and often have a tendency to make the healer believe they are more special than anyone else. One can get a false sense of power from this plane.

- Healers who still have Fourth-Plane commitments believe they cannot work on themselves. This is also a criterion of the Fifth Plane.

Energy test for:

'I have to suffer to learn.'

'I learn the hard way.'

'I am expected to suffer.'

'The more I suffer, the closer I am to God.'

'I have to go through a death door or die to grow spiritually.'

Replace with:

'I learn without suffering,'

'I learn from the Creator.'

'I learn with ease and freedom.'

'I know the definition of dedication from the Creator of All That Is.'

'I am always connected to the Creator of All That Is.'

'I grow spiritually through the Creator of All That Is.'

SPIRITS AND ANCESTORS

WAYWARD SPIRITS

It is on this plane that we learn how to send uncontrolled energies or 'wayward' spirits to God's light. Wayward spirits, you will recall, are those who are temporarily trapped between the Third and Fourth Plane, afraid to go to light. They can be spirits who simply do not believe in the light, or who have committed suicide or had other traumatic deaths, or who are afraid to go to the light because they are afraid they will become the light. They can be sent to the Creator's light by using a simple exercise. To recap:

THE PROCESS FOR WAYWARD SPIRITS

1. Centre yourself in your heart and visualize going down into Mother Earth, which is a part of All That Is.

2. Visualize bringing up energy through your feet, opening each chakra to the crown chakra. In a beautiful ball of light, go out to the universe.

3. Go beyond the universe, past the white lights, past the dark light, past the white light, past the jelly-like substance that is the Laws, into a pearly iridescent white light, into the Seventh Plane of Existence.

4. Make the command: *'Creator of All That Is, it is commanded that all wayward spirits around [person's name] be sent to God's light to be transformed. Thank you! It is done. It is done. It is done.'*

5. Move over to the person's crown. Witness the wayward spirits being sent to the Creator's light using your connection or the client's connection to Source. Be sure you follow them all the way to the Creator's light, as they will attempt to escape.

6. As soon as the process is finished, rinse yourself off and put yourself back into your space. Go into the Earth, pull Earth energy up through all your chakras to your crown chakra and make an energy break.

CONNECTING TO YOUR ANCESTORS

One thing that is useful when using the Fourth Plane is connecting to your ancestors or those of your clients. When you are doing this on behalf of a client, it is likely that they will have unfinished programmes connected to the deceased. This process will assist them to complete these.

In this process you will command that someone the client has previously known will come and visit them. Ask the client the name of the deceased person they would like to talk to and call to that spirit. You will be the spokesperson for the spirit without permitting it to enter your body.

Bear in mind that the spirits that are held on this plane are not necessarily enlightened beings and will come to you in much the same *persona* that they had when alive. They will even retain some physical attributes, such as sexual attraction and many other passions. So it is recommended that the client call on someone that they are fond of.

You can speak to animals that have gone as well. Trust in the first thoughts and voices that come into your mind.

Other reasons for this exercise are to show you that you can speak to ancestor spirits or friends and allow you to get a feel of what the different dimensions are like. It shows you the difference between these levels and Creation, as well as what a divine thought form feels like as opposed to one of your own or those of other people.

THE PROCESS FOR CONNECTING TO YOUR ANCESTORS

Prior to beginning this exercise, ask permission to see and speak to the person's ancestor spirit. Ask for the spirit's name.

1. Ground and centre yourself.

2. Begin by sending your consciousness down into the centre of Mother Earth, which is a part of All That Is. Bring the energy up through your feet, into your body and up through all the chakras. Go up through your crown chakra and raise and project your consciousness out in a beautiful ball of light past the stars to the universe.

3. Go beyond the universe, past the white lights, past the dark light, past the white light, past the jelly-like substance that is the Laws, into a pearly iridescent white light, into the Seventh Plane of Existence.

4. Gather unconditional love and make the command: *'Creator, it is commanded to see and speak with [name of spirit] at this time. Thank you. It is done. It is done. It is done.'*

5. Go directly to the person's space and look over their shoulders. Call the ancestor spirit or animal spirit in and wait for them to show themselves.

6. You may see balls of light. Ask the spirit the client's questions and share with them the responses received. Trust in the first thoughts that come into your mind.

7. When you have finished, rinse yourself off, put yourself back in your space and make an energy break.

13

THE THIRD PLANE

This is the plane of our everyday reality. In part, we have created it for our use. It is on this plane that we have the challenge of being governed by emotions, instinctual desires and passions and the reality of being in the human body. Our consciousness mostly stays on this plane, even though we are deeply connected to all the planes.

In the creation of our own reality, we have made programmes, thought forms and collective consciousness in and throughout the Third Plane that keep us in this plane. This means that some of our physical, mental and spiritual capabilities are blocked. In order to break free of the chains that bind us, we must concentrate upon the joy of life instead of fear, anger and hatred. Since the ego lives on and in the Third Plane, we must control the negative ego in ourselves. How we balance our emotions will dictate how well we are able to break free from the Third Plane and access and move freely through all the other planes to create health and manifest other changes in this reality.

We often forget we are here to experience *joy*, to breathe, to live in this wonderful way. Our lungs celebrate each time we take a breath of air. Do we stop to feel this celebration? We should remind ourselves that this is a wonderful plane to exist in. The cells in the body are working so very hard to give us this life experience. The liver and other organs are working overtime for us to be here. Since physical exercise keeps our body grounded and enjoying the Third Plane, it is important to have a regular exercise routine to follow in order to celebrate the human body.

We are here to learn as spiritual beings, and some of us still learn from pain and suffering. This is one of our spiritual challenges on this plane: to learn without suffering and through joy. It is our responsibility to accept that the human body is a wonderful place to live in.

Humans are in fact walking miracles! We learn to manipulate our body, use our brain, control our limbs, communicate our ideas and act upon our thoughts, ideas and dreams. This is the plane of imagination, problem-solving, fight or flight.

LIVING ON ALL THE PLANES

We may think that we're physically on the Third Plane of Existence, but we actually exist on all of the seven planes. In reality, as already explained, humans of the Third Plane are children of the Fifth Plane. Some of us have some conscious recollection of this. In fact, many religions are based upon this thought. This explains why many people believe they are 'children of God', because we all have a heavenly father and mother on the Fifth Plane, yet are still connected to the All That Is.

Our spiritual parents give us encouragement, compassion and advice. Each one of us has these incredible beings leading us along the path to enlightenment. They are high masters from the Fifth Plane. To meet your spiritual parents it is best to go through the Creator of All That Is of the Seventh Plane. This is because once you have been purified in the essence of the Creator you will be better able to communicate clearly with them.

Remember that many of the people here on Earth now are actually masters from the Fifth Plane who have come here to help their Third-Plane students/children home to the Fifth Plane. If you often feel as though you do not belong here on Earth, that the Earth is too harsh, that the people are cruel, and you feel incredibly homesick and miss your spiritual family, then you may be a Fifth-Plane master. If you know you have incredible abilities and a strong connection to the Creator, you may be a master waking up to help the Earth. The masters of the Fifth Plane that have come here can easily remember how to direct their mind. All of the high Fifth-Plane masters use the Seventh Plane to create.

HEALING FROM THE THIRD PLANE

Remember that healers working from the Third Plane often get caught up in the drama of this plane and believe that some things are incurable because of group consciousness. They are governed by time, and also often get involved in the dualism of good and evil, a Fifth-Plane energy, instead of the Seventh-Plane energy of love and All That Is.

On the Third Plane it is the removal and replacement of belief systems as well as the addition of *feelings* that gives us the opening to the vibrations of the other planes of existence. It is then that we are released from karmic influences. The more beliefs that are changed, the faster we are able to access the other planes.

Healers on the Third Plane often use the other planes instinctively. For example, if a surgeon carries out an operation and uses a scalpel, then they are accessing the First and Third Plane of Existence. They are the representation of the Third Plane and the scalpel is of the First Plane. Other planes are accessed in the surgical process, such as the Laws of the Universe on the Sixth Plane.

An example of this would be in the very thought process of the surgery: 'If I cut this tumour from this organ in the correct way, it follows that the tissues will separate in such a way as to remove the tumour without causing further damage and be of benefit to this person.' In this process the surgeon is instinctively accessing the Law of Cause and Effect. While all this is going on, the brain sends neurons through the system to move the surgeon's hands and at the same time regulates the many systems in their body. This is an amazing feat of God's engineering. And while the surgeon is saving the person's life, the other members of the theatre staff are unwittingly accessing the Second Plane by administering the penicillin and the IV drip to the person.

It is on the Third Plane that you can communicate with and heal animals, as outlined in *ThetaHealing*.

The foremost thing to remember about the Third-Plane reality is that this plane is an *illusion* and is not real. The only thing real about *any* of it is what you create in it.

14

THE SECOND PLANE

My first experience of the Second Plane of Existence was in northern Idaho in the early years of ThetaHealing.

In these years, most of my seminars were arranged by people who had had readings from me. One of my clients, Gretchen, had co-ordinated a class in the town of Sandpoint, Idaho. I found northern Idaho to be an intensely beautiful place, with deep forests, towering mountains, rushing rivers and crystal-clear lakes. Located in the Idaho panhandle with Montana on one side and Washington on the other, it is wild, primal and permeated with the energy of the natural world. Sandpoint is right in the middle of this area and was the stage for one of my first DNA 1 classes. This was a two-day course, so Guy and I went to stay there for two nights.

Gretchen had arranged for us to stay with one of the students named Peggy. She lived above the town in the mountains in a beautiful log cabin crafted of rough-hewn lumber. Needless to say, it had a rustic beauty that appealed to Guy. To me, it was like a gingerbread house from a fairy tale.

As it turned out, Peggy was a believer in the little people, the fairies. She unabashedly told us that one of her ambitions in life was to see a fairy in the flesh, but so far she had been unsuccessful. She was a spunky person with a lot of personality and told us she could sense nature spirits around her place and was a little put out that they did not appear for her.

At this time in my life, I didn't have a lot of credence in fairies. I had seen ghosts and apparitions, but I had never seen fairies, and I raised a skeptical Mr Spock eyebrow at Peggy. I thought that she was a little wishful, and also rather venomous in her behaviour towards these fairies who would not appear for her.

I had to admit that the place had a magical essence to it, the sort of timelessness that you only encounter in certain areas. It was early summer and there were flowers in bloom in the garden. As darkness fell on the mountains, the evening began to sing its song, and Guy and I went to sleep to be ready for the first day of the seminar the next day.

The next morning Peggy woke us up and I reluctantly rolled out of bed to shower. I didn't know it, but I was about to have an experience that would shake my belief system like a tree in a gale.

I was in the shower stall, shaving my legs, as I regularly do, minding my own business, when all of a sudden three little creatures flew in through the small open window. At first I thought that they were hummingbirds. But they looked like tiny people with wings. They spun about my body in a swirl of curious energy. I stood frozen in mid-motion with a shaver in one hand, so full of surprise that I couldn't move.

The beings weren't wearing any clothes and they all appeared to be female. They looked like nine-year-old girls with wings. Their skin colour was tan and they had long hair in different hues of brown. Their eyes sparkled at me as they flew. Their wings were moving almost too fast to see. One of them hovered at eye level with me and I could hear a voice in my head that I somehow knew came from all of the creatures at once.

'What are you doing?'

The answer came to me automatically: 'I'm shaving the hair on my legs.'

There was a brief pause and then the musical voice chimed in my head again: '*Why* are you shaving the hair on your legs?'

I told them, 'I'm a human woman. I have to shave the hair on my legs.'

They burst into laughter that sounded like tinkling bells in my head and rolled around in mid-air, pointing at me. With a *poof!*, one of them grew long hair on her legs. The others laughed at her, turning in circles with hilarity.

Suddenly they all flew out of the window into the forest and in a wink were gone.

I felt unhinged! I thought I was losing my mind. I ran into the bedroom in tears and in a rush I told Guy about my experience. I asked him if I was going crazy.

Guy looked at me calmly and said, 'Vianna, you have just seen fairies.'

I looked at him blankly.

'You know, *nature spirits*. Many people have seen them, but it is uncommon. They are attached to places where flowers grow and the trees are thick, and sometimes to old sacred sites. They have been seen on every continent in some form or another. The Native Americans have many legends about them that are somewhat similar to those of Ireland. Since you are intuitive, it is easier for you to see them than most people. You are like a bridge between humans and the fairy world. So, calm down! You're not going crazy, you're just able to see them.'

As I listened to him, I began to compose myself. Bit by bit, I pulled myself together and began to get dressed for the day, all the while looking out the corners of my eyes, fearful of seeing some unwanted apparition.

We went down to the kitchen for breakfast and I told Peggy what I had seen, thinking she would be happy to hear about it. I was wrong. She was very upset, because she had been trying to see fairies for over 20 years and had been putting out bowls of milk and honey as offerings to them for a long time and then I had come to her home and in a few hours they had appeared to me! She was a little grumpy about the whole thing, and continued to be so for the two days that we stayed with her.

Her morning had already been complicated by another incident. Bears had been visiting her in the night and it seems that one had made a near-impossible climb onto the back deck to make a raid on the bird feeder. The feeder had been destroyed and seed was everywhere. Peggy was intensely frustrated by this, and the swarms of birds weren't very happy either. The hungry bear had also left a smelly calling card on the deck as a lasting reminder.

Two days later we had finished the seminar. As we drove away from Peggy's home, I said goodbye to the little fairy house and to the little people who in a brief instant had shocked me, stolen my innocence and given it back again.

This incident with the fairies changed my concept of reality forever. It opened me to the possibilities of the Second Plane of Existence.

❖❖❖❖❖

My experience with the people from the Second Plane wasn't over. It wasn't long after my meeting with the little fairies in the shower that I was visited again. I was on my way home from a seminar in St George, Utah. For those of you who have not seen this area, it is a very beautiful place. The Utah desert is a wild area with sweeping blood-red vistas. There are endless juniper forests, majestic crimson mountains that change with the light, and the river bottom of the Virgin river with willows and cottonwood trees that are inviting in the desert heat.

On this day I felt compelled to wash the crystals that I had just acquired. Whenever I get new crystals it is a kind of ritual for me to wash off any ghost imprints from them in a rushing stream. I saw a likely spot in the river and stopped off to cleanse them close to the entrance of Zion National Park.

I walked down to the river and was bent down washing my crystals when all of a sudden two fairies materialized from the brush and flew around my head. They were wearing clothing made of autumn leaves, and their little wings were beating so fast they were hard to see, much like those of a hummingbird. One was a boy and the other a girl. My first thought was, 'Oh! They come in boys.'

The little boy fairy flew up close to my face and said, 'Give it to me!' indicating the crystal in my hand.

I was instantly irritated. I told him, 'No! You can't have it.'

The boy fairy was insistent and became aggressive, flying around my head and pulling at my hair. He screamed at me, 'Give it to me!'

'No!' I screamed back as I ducked to avoid his attack.

For his small size he was incredibly strong. He began to fly at me, pushing me in an attempt to dump me in the river behind me. He was tiny, but so powerful! I began to thrash about as I swatted at him. I began to be frightened that I would fall into the water, since at this time of the year it was running deep and cold.

Then, out of the corner of my eye, I saw a movement behind me. All of a sudden a tall woman came rising out of the river, a vision of flowing liquid beauty. She pointed at the boy fairy and her eyes flashed with an electric blue, projecting annoyance at him. She said, 'Leave her alone!'

Both of the fairies were terrified. With little squeals, they went flying off. Soon they had disappeared.

Grateful to the beautiful water elemental who had saved me, I picked up my crystals and beat a hasty retreat to my car, where I collapsed onto the seat and began to cry. My husband comforted me. When I felt better, we drove home.

This incident doesn't mean that all fairies are bad. They can be mischievous, but can become good friends if we have proper respect for them. However, the energies of this plane are powerful, perhaps even intense at times. This is why our connection to the Creator of All That Is of the Seventh Plane of Existence must be clear. Though I didn't know it at the time, all I needed to do when the little fairy attacked me was to connect to the Creator and, through the Creator, command that he go away.

Since that time I have had many other meetings with the blessed people, and on more than one continent. But those are other stories.

NATURE SPIRITS – ELEMENTALS

Because of the spiritual evolution of humankind, the veils are now becoming thin between the planes. It is much easier for people to see through them than ever before. The veil between the Second and Third Plane is becoming particularly thin. Because of this opening in the space-time continuum, greater numbers of people are witnessing fairies.

I like to call them elementals, and make no mistake, they are not human in *any way*. They can control the rate of their molecular vibration to take on the different forms of the elements – earth, air, water and fire. They can become a wisp of wind, the babble of the rushing stream, the earth beneath our feet or even the fire of lightning. They can merge with plants, become a being of liquid or air or take a solid form. It is when they choose to take solid form that we see them in their myriad of different shapes and sizes as fairies.

Anyone who has a special love for trees or plants will have an intrinsic connection to elementals, and some elementals have learned to communicate with humans. For some humans this is good; for others, it may not be. Fairies do not always act with benevolence towards humans. They do not like to be ordered around, but can be utilized if approached in the correct fashion.

In one of my classes in Australia, someone came up with an interesting point: they found that anytime they connected to the elementals and asked them for help, the elementals expected a gift in return. So if you find your keys missing from your purse, or some other article has gone, this can be the fairies exacting their just due.

If you should decide to open your home up to fairies, then you should do so from the Seventh Plane of Existence. In this way, human and elemental will enhance each other's lives and not be at odds. Through the Seventh Plane, the energies of the Second and Third Plane will work together.

Here is a list of guidelines to follow:

- Always go to the Seventh Plane before talking to elementals.

- Never go anywhere with an elemental until you've gone up to the Seventh Plane first.

- Never ask a favour of an elemental, because they expect an exchange of energy and will take shiny objects without permission, feeling completely justified.

- Elementals are not gods.

- Elementals respect you more if you respect yourself.

- Elementals only show themselves to those who are pure in heart.

- You don't have to believe in elementals in order to see one.

- Elementals will only show themselves if they know they are in no danger.

- Elementals are enchanted by humans' singing and laughter. (The songs must be in tune.)

- Elementals love art. They love watching people paint pictures.

Elementals have a tendency to love shiny things, because of the refractive index of light that they create, much in the same way that we appreciate a sparkling diamond. There are elementals that are attracted to beautiful crystal formations such as quartzite and amethyst. An energy is created when light hits a crystal formation. This fusion of light and crystal, this *luminescence*, is soma to the elementals. This is why they are drawn to crystals.

Because the veils are beginning to drop between the planes of existence, I believe that some elementals have come to inhabit human form. We have all seen people who act as though they are elves or fairies. It almost seems as though they are evolving or devolving into fairies. I believe that many elementals do this just to have the experience of the Third Plane. Many of them are here on the Third Plane to protect the elementals and their habitat. They are often environmentalists and naturalists.

LIVING IN HARMONY WITH THE SECOND PLANE OF EXISTENCE

As a species, we have developed a symbiotic relationship with plants. They use us to propagate and spread themselves and are in turn, indispensable to our survival. Plants perform the miracle of photosynthesis, the sacred creation of blessed sunlight into pure energy for us to consume. We thrive on this energy and plant the seeds in the earth to begin the cycle anew.

Plants are highly evolved; they live from light and minerals and, on the whole, use no other living organic material. All plant beings have their own consciousness. Along with the earth and air spirits, they act out the sacred dance of interconnection between the First and Third Planes of Existence, transmigrating the life force for the animals to utilize.

Plants and trees are some of the most evolved and sacred of God's creatures. In the cycle of birth and death, they gather nutrients through their roots from Mother Earth and are still returning the same nutrients long after they die. They follow the Nature's sacred cycle and only compete to live, not destroy. While only consuming sunlight, air and soil to sustain themselves, they provide nourishment and shelter for many other living beings.

Love, joy, happiness and respect are the keys to truly understanding plants and trees. When using them to heal, whether home-grown or wild-crafted, we should remember to harvest whatever is necessary with respect. Remember to go up out of your space and connect to the Creator, then ask the plants' permission to harvest them. They should speak back to you and will direct you to the plants that will suit the intended use. As you harvest the plant, be connected to the Creator, go back to the time the plant was a seed and pour love and blessing into the seed as you watch it grow into its present form.

The elemental kingdom is intertwined with the plants and also with the pure essence of light. Therefore the Second Plane of Existence transmutes the light of the sun and directs this energy throughout all the planes to create life.

Sunlight is the essence of life. All the creatures of the Earth need it to live. Everything on this planet is based upon the fire of light and we assimilate it by consuming plants. The actual life force, the *light* that is within in the plant, is what is important to the human body. This utilization of light is a way for us to stay connected to all the planes of existence.

Healers using the Second Plane of Existence understand how to use herbs and vitamins in order to achieve health. Healing from this plane requires time and persistence. Healers working with this plane require an extensive knowledge of plants and reactions to medicines. Without this knowledge, there is a risk to the client. But there is an organic combination of plants for every illness.

As already mentioned, when using herbs or other plants to heal, the proper procedure is to bless the plant from the seed to the present. Similarly, when you buy herbs, vitamins or food, remember to ask the Creator of All That Is if they are for your highest good. You can determine this by connecting to the Creator while holding the product.

Since everything has a consciousness and we absorb this essence when we consume it, we need to bless all the food we eat. If it has not been treated with the respect it deserves, the benefits will be reduced. Remember that genetically altered food has a consciousness that is perhaps not for our best. If there is a question about the essence of any food, go back and bless it from its origin.

MEET THE SECOND PLANE OF EXISTENCE
THROUGH THE SEVENTH PLANE

The best way to experience the Second Plane of Existence is to go to the Seventh Plane of Existence first and then to go to the Second Plane.

Plants are very sensitive and if you push your thoughts towards them too forcefully, they can literally die. This exercise is designed to demonstrate how sensitive plants are, to teach you how to move gently in and out of another being's living space undetected and to give you the chance to practise your scanning abilities. This will sharpen your skills, as well as your discernment.

MEET A PLANT

1. Ground and centre yourself.

2. Begin by sending your consciousness down into the centre of Mother Earth, which is a part of All That Is. Bring the energy up through your

feet, into your body and up through all the chakras. Go up through your crown chakra in a beautiful ball of light, out past the stars to the universe.

3. Go beyond the universe, past the white lights, past the dark light, past the white light, past the jelly-like substance that is the Laws, into a pearly iridescent white light, into the Seventh Plane of Existence.

4. Gather unconditional love and make the command to the Creator of All That Is: *'Creator of All That Is, a scan of this plant is commanded. Show me what I need to see. Thank you. It is done. It is done. It is done.'*

5. Go to the plant as gently as a feather on a summer breeze. Now, imagine going gently into the plant, taking a quick look and then moving out of its space. Remember, if you go in with too much force, you can actually cause harm to the plant.

6. Rinse yourself off, ground yourself, go back into your space and make an energy break.

15

THE FIRST PLANE

When I was 29 years old I heard of a rock and crystal peddler who had come to town. He was selling his wares in a booth at the local mall. I have always loved the essence and vibration of rocks, minerals and crystals. In south-eastern Idaho the metaphysical community is always on the lookout for good deals on crystals with high energy. So when I heard about this peddler I was curious to see what he had. I went to the mall on an adventure to find the perfect crystal.

The rock peddler was a man I came to know as Chuck. At that time he was about 55 years old. He was part Native American and had long hair. As I was viewing what he had on his little cart, I spied a little crystal in the shape of a pyramid hanging on a silver chain and immediately fell in love with it.

At that time in my life I was having a very difficult time making ends meet. I was studying and had very little to live on. In spite of this, I pulled $15 out of my pocket to buy the necklace.

Chuck looked at me and said, 'You don't want that necklace.'

This perplexed and annoyed me a little. I said, 'Yes, I do.'

He replied, 'No, you don't. You want this one, or perhaps this one.'

The necklaces that he indicated were much more intricate and better designed than the crystal I had chosen, but I said, 'No, neither of those is the one I want. I want this one,' indicating the little crystal the shape of the pyramid.

I handed over my money, and as I did so, Chuck said, 'Well, if you buy this necklace, you have to have this as well.'

From under the edge of the cart he pulled out a black rock with shiny little facets on it. It was absolutely stunning.

I looked at him and asked him, 'How much is it?'

He said, 'How much do you have?'

'I have $8.'

He looked at me and smiled and said, 'Then for today, it's $8, and handed me the stone.

From that day my life began to change. From the moment I brought the stone home, I began to become much more psychically attuned to things around me.

I must admit I was profoundly taken with the stone. It was almost as though it would talk to me. Each time I held it, I found that I could focus my intuitive abilities more easily.

This piqued my curiosity to find out what the stone was. I asked many people, but no one could tell me. Finally, about a year and a half later, I went to a rock and mineral show. I took the crystal with me and showed it to one of the vendors there. He instantly offered to buy it for $80, but he wouldn't tell me what it was. I declined his offer and took it to another vendor. He told me that it was a melanite crystal, one of the andradite garnet mineral families. I was unfamiliar with the term and said, 'Excuse me?'

The man said, 'Darling, that is what some in the trade call a black ruby. I have never seen one that size in my life. They usually only occur in much smaller single square faucets and are rarely clumped together like this. I don't know how much this particular specimen is worth, but if I were you I would hold on to it.'

Ever since that day, my little 'black ruby' has been one of my special crystals. Upon experimentation I found that it was one of the very few stones that could hold energy under a pyramid. Most stones will become as cold as ice under a pyramid. The only stones I have found that hold their energy are rutilated quartz and my black ruby.

I found that my black ruby held many mystical and magical secrets. The most important aspect of it was that it woke up my intuitive senses. To this day it is one of my sweetest, most precious friends out of all my crystals.

This was how I first became intimately acquainted with the First Plane of Existence and the power of crystals.

THE LIFE OF THE FIRST PLANE OF EXISTENCE

From the First Plane, we learn that non-organic life has life and a consciousness of its own. Mother Earth herself is a giant energy field or giant spirit. Every piece of Earth, from the smallest crystal to the largest mountain, has its own peculiar spirit. Even though as humans we do not see these spirits move, they still have their own life force.

To have life, as science understands it, you need to have a carbon atom to make a carbon molecular structure. On the First Plane, there is life that is beyond anything that we understand as carbon based. This plane is composed of non-organic material.

This non-organic life is all around us. Mother Earth cradles the rocks, and within the rocks are minerals. The minerals are composed of calcium, magnesium and selenium, which we need traces of to survive. In fact, we are composed of these very minerals, along with water. This is the base of molecular structure.

MINERALS

Minerals have two general functions: building and regulating. Their building functions affect our bones, teeth and all soft tissues. Their regulating functions include a wide variety of systems, such as the beating of our heart, the clotting of our blood, maintaining nerve responses and transporting oxygen from our lungs to the tissues. Along with protein, carbohydrates, fats, water and vitamins, we must have minerals to build a strong body and to carry on all its delicate life processes. If we were not in constant concert with the First Plane via minerals, we would turn into water, because it is the minerals that, to a large degree, comprise our bones and tissues.

As health-conscious people we all know it is necessary to provide our body with proper vitamins and minerals, but very few of us understand why. While vitamins and minerals are very different, the body must have both. One obvious difference is that vitamins contain carbon and are considered to be organic substances. Minerals are deficient in carbon and therefore are classified as inorganic substances.

Both have important roles. The body can continue to function without getting the recommended daily allowance of some vitamins, but a mineral deficiency can have disastrous effects. For instance, in order to make the haemoglobin found in red blood cells, the body needs iron. In order to build strong teeth and bones, it needs calcium. Calcium is also vital for the proper functioning of the kidneys, muscles and nerves. Without sufficient levels of iodine, the thyroid gland cannot produce energy. Manganese, selenium and zinc are antioxidants and some of their tasks include helping to heal wounds, helping the skeletal system to develop properly and shielding cell membranes.

The body needs two classes of minerals: major minerals and trace minerals. The difference between them has to do with the amount needed. It is necessary for the body to have a minimum of 100 milligrams per day of the major minerals to carry out its functions properly. In the case of trace minerals, less than 100 milligrams is required per day.

The Seven Major Minerals

calcium

chloride

magnesium

phosphorus

potassium

sodium

sulphur

The Trace Minerals

chromium

copper

fluoride

iodine

iron

manganese

molybdenum

selenium

zinc

If there is a lack of minerals, there is a lack of support.

Mineral Sources

We get our minerals from the foods we eat. How does this happen? Minerals make their way into our body by means of the foods that grow from the ground and the animals that live off the land. Fruit, vegetables, lean meat, poultry, dairy products, grains and legumes are some of the primary sources of the minerals our body needs to thrive. Processed foods are low in minerals and people who do not have a proper diet often suffer from diseases directly attributable to vitamin- and mineral-related deficiencies.

Of all the deficiencies I have encountered in clients, few are as prevalent as deficiencies of calcium and magnesium. Very few people that I have looked at actually have enough calcium in their body.

I believe that mineral deficiency is an underlying cause of many modern illnesses. Due to the depletion of our soils, minerals are no longer as available to us as they once were.

Because excessive amounts of some minerals inside the body can have a toxic effect, there is controversy surrounding mineral supplementation. We should do our best to meet our daily mineral requirements from food, but a suggestion for proper absorption of supplemental minerals is to take a *chelated* mineral. It is easier for these to get into the bloodstream and be absorbed through the walls of the cells. Absorption of non-chelated minerals is more difficult.

The Theta practitioner learns to see the deficiencies of minerals in the body psychically and can psychically produce different minerals in the body if mastership is accomplished on this plane.

This is the plane of the mastership of the *alchemist* and the knowledge of transmutation of minerals from one form to another. Because telekinesis is moving non-organic matter, the power of telekinesis is learned here, too, with an equation of the Seventh and Sixth Plane. The ability to move objects or to bend spoons with the electromagnetic power of the mind is held on this plane.

When a healer uses minerals they are using this plane of existence. There is a mineral for every sickness. Healings using crystals are also from this plane of existence. This requires time and energy.

CRYSTALS AND HEALING STONES

The First Plane of Existence teaches us how to connect with rocks, gemstones, minerals, the air that we breathe and the Earth beneath us. Ultimately, the purpose is to foster a relationship of respect and honour for our planet Earth, which is a part of All That Is.

The First Plane has its own peculiar consciousness. Even though you don't see with the naked eye minerals broken down into their composite elements and only see them as solids, understand that they are still moving, only extremely slowly. I am telling you that there is a consciousness in everything that is. Just as you and I have one, so do non-organic life forms.

Ancient peoples around the world connected with the energies of crystals and minerals and gave these powers names, such as the 'stone people'. They were aware of the different attributes of crystals and minerals and how these could be used to enhance a person's abilities as well as open doorways to the powers of the other planes of existence. Many doorways to the other planes can be accessed using the energies of crystals and minerals. One may use crystals for connecting to ancestral DNA memory in an equation with the Third Plane of Existence, for example.

An intuitive person can learn the hidden language of minerals and crystals and uncover the knowledge held in the records stored in them. This is why they are often drawn to a particular stone or crystal. That stone is calling to them because it is appropriate for them at that time in their life, for a mystical or physical reason, or because it needs them in some way.

Did you know that modern science has discovered that the hormones in the body are actually crystalline in structure? The way that they are released and sent through the body is almost identical to the growth of crystals.

It is also interesting to note that it is thought that most gemstones were created over 200 million years ago. Created by hydrothermal and magmatic cycles deep in the Earth, many of the stones that we know and treasure have undergone a long and magnificent journey before becoming our friends in healing, jewellery and centrepieces. Their incredible age, accompanied by their beauty, gives us a connection to the serenity and mystery of the world we live in.

Most stones, semi-precious or otherwise, come with their own traditions. Some people use them for *feng shui* and to transmute negative energy. A true master of gemstones only uses them to enhance things and never gives the power of decision-making over to the stones themselves. Remember, you really need no help or tools in commanding a healing; you simply need to go to the Creator of All That Is. You are learning about crystals so that you can communicate with those people who still think they need these tools. It's also fun to know many things and how to work with each plane of existence, but don't get too caught up in this brain candy. The Creator is all you need.

The lesson of crystal healing is discernment. Crystals only enhance the energy of the bearer that wears and uses them, just as electrical equipment is enhanced by electricity. You must understand that stones actually work with the electricity of your own mind and body. As your energy vibration changes, you are drawn to different stones with different attributes.

If you wear or carry rocks and crystals, you will find that they do have special qualities, which the Creator has endowed them with. Learn the qualities of the rocks around you; they will aid you in realizing that you are not separate from All That Is.

HOW TO TAKE CARE OF CRYSTALS

To care for crystals, wash them by sitting them in sunlight, moonlight or sea salt or washing them in ocean water, stream water and even by toning them with tuning forks or bells.

Remember that some crystals are delicate and should not be washed.

The best and most accurate way to clean crystals is by going up to the Creator of All That Is and commanding them to be cleaned.

HEALING CRYSTALS

Stones have many purposes. Here is a list of stones and some of their purposes. Remember that not all books pertaining to crystals and their metaphysical attributes will agree with one another.

Agate: Grounding stones that bring emotional, physical and mental balance and help overcome negativity, bitterness and inner anger.

Blue lace agate: Has a calming, peaceful, healing effect.

Fire agate: A protective stone.

Moss agate: Refreshes the soul and wakes us up to the beauty around us. It lessens pain and boosts the lymph system and the immune system.

Amber: This not a crystal, but petrified tree sap, so a fossil. It has the power to draw out disease. It also gets rid of stress and is a great healing stone for all of the internal organs. It also triggers past-life memories, whether our own or genetic.

Amethyst: Increases clairvoyance and divine connection and brings common sense.

Aquamarine: Stimulates release and change, gives courage and helps intuition and clairvoyance.

Aventurine: Brings adventure into our life and helps us create our dreams.

Azurite: Increases intuition amazingly and clears the chakras. It was extremely valued by the ancients, even more than lapis.

Bloodstone: The legend is that Christ bled on certain stones, and those few stones are called bloodstones. They give us courage and wake us up to our Christ energy.

Carnelian: Gives courage, promotes positive life choices, dispels apathy and motivates success in business and other activities.

Charoite: Connects us to our true divine purpose. Aids in coping with change as we move to a higher spiritual level. Transmutes negative energy into healing, converts disease into health and brings powerful dreams.

Citrine: Brings prosperity and abundance.

Dioptase: Heals and comforts the heart and brings in forgiveness. Helps us live in the present moment.

Emerald: Converts negative energy into positive and brings patience. A major heart centre stone, it brings protection and healing.

Fluorite: It is excellent for learning, has an emotionally stabilizing effect and is good for infections.

Garnet: Brings prosperity and passion, inspires love and regenerates the body.

Haematite: Protection of the warrior, grounding. It is used in the treatment of arthritis and high blood pressure.

Jade: Protection, healing; will absorb all negative energies and shatter when it is full. It never has to be washed. It doesn't hold any ghost imprints.

Jasper: All jasper has healing properties.

Madagascar jasper: A rare and beautiful stone found only in one place in the world.

Kyanite: An amazing healing stone that never has to be washed. It takes pain away. It does not keep any negative energy but transmutes it instantly. Instills compassion and lowers blood pressure.

Labradorite: Stone of mystics, this converts negative energy into positive energy. It always connects us to true magic.

Lapis lazuli: An ancient stone used to send telepathic messages and to wake up and enhance psychic abilities.

Larimar: Nurturing, it brings clarity and constructive thought.

Malachite: Used for protection, courage and to strengthen the will. It will shatter when we are in danger.

Moldavite: Used for transformation. Speeds up what we're already creating in our life. Avoid it if your world is already fast-paced.

Moonstone: Brings our soul mate to us, encourages lucid dreaming, enhances psychic abilities and calms emotions.

Obsidian: Offers protection against negative thought forms and spells.

Onyx: Healing and protection.

Black onyx: Protection against negative energies. Helps the wearer to dissolve an unwanted relationship.

Opal: It was once said that if you wear an opal, you can wear no other stone. This was a myth made up by diamond sellers, because opals were becoming more popular than diamonds. Opal brings us to our true abilities. It is a water stone; it loves water. Wear it with anything you like.

Petrified wood: New beginnings and protection.

Pyrite: A male stone, it wakes up our male attributes.

Quartz: Brings clarity, healing.

Rose quartz: Used for love and heart healing.

Smoky quartz: Used for protection from negative energy and for grounding.

Rhodochrosite: Brings love and teaches us to love ourselves and nurture ourselves.

Seraphinite: Sister of charoite, it brings spiritual connection.

Sodalite: Starts us on our journey.

Tiger's eye: Helps our ability to see the future. Integrates both sides of the brain. Use it to accomplish goals.

Topaz: Magnifies our intention, converts negative energy into positive energy.

Yellow topaz: Brings money.

Tourmaline: Enhances the energies of a quartz crystal. It's ten times stronger than quartz. It is a better conductor than quartz, and is used in telescopes, televisions and other electrical appliances. Ancients believed that it helped them receive clearer messages, helped to send thoughts and increased their psychic abilities. It brings inner peace.

Black tourmaline: Purifies the body.

Turquoise: Blue turquoise is healing; it takes the pain out of arthritis.

16

HEALING WITH THE PLANES

When a person first begins to use the Theta technique they connect to different planes' power and are unfamiliar as to which one that they are using. Since all the planes are connected to the divine, it can be easy to become confused. The best way to learn about healing with the planes is to connect to them and experience them. Always go to the Seventh Plane first so you are not bound by the rules and commitments of the other planes.

Remember that each of the planes has a cure for every emotion or disease in the body. On the First Plane, for example, there is one chemical combination or one mineral combination to repair every disease. This combination has the same vibration as the programme that may contributing to the disease, and so can replace it.

Correspondingly, there is one herb or vitamin, or possibly several herbs or vitamins, from the Second Plane of Existence to heal every disease. We live in the Third Plane of proteins, which means there is an amino acid combination that will contribute to healing any sickness. On the Fourth Plane of Existence there are the right carbohydrates to create healing energy for the body, and shamans use the plants and spiritual ancestors to heal. On the Fifth Plane of Existence, angels and your heavenly parents can heal your body. You may have to trade for the healing, you may have to make changes for it, but in the process, you will clean up your belief systems. The essences of the Fourth and Fifth Planes will usually make you promise to do certain things *that will change your vibration*.

Once connected to the Sixth Plane of Existence, you will hear music and tones. This means that on this plane we use vibrations to heal.

When it comes down to it, all of the planes are about *light*, about *vibration*. With the right mineral, there is the right vibration; with the right plant, there is the right vibration. All of these physical things that you consume are the same vibration as the belief work that you do, and will heal the body. A herb that acts as an antibiotic has the right vibration to heal you from a bacterium, for example, and this means it also has the right vibration to heal you from the guilt programme that draws the bacterium. This is because every plane of existence has the right answer. There is the right mineral, the right vitamin, the right protein, the right programme and the right feeling.

It is possible that belief work will do the same thing as every cure from every plane of existence. So what do you do if you have a client who really doesn't believe in belief work? Well, you won't, because your clients are coming to you for the belief work. I recommend that they are downloaded with all the programmes from the feeling work in this book (*see pages 33–70*). Then it will be possible for them to let go of everything that doesn't serve them easily and quickly.

True healing comes to everyone who finally learns what it feels like to have love. The friction between fear and love exists on the Fifth Plane and here on the Third. I believe that once there is no fear, once again it will be a question of 'It just is', as it is on the Seventh Plane. But you can figure that out for yourself now that you understand how the planes of existence work.

THE STRUCTURE OF LIFE OF THE PLANES

To briefly recap information given in *ThetaHealing*, the human body is made up of five different compounds: lipids, carbohydrates, proteins, adenosine triphosphate (ATP), or energy, and nucleic acid, which is DNA. These five components are the staff of life that interconnect you and make you a Seventh-Plane being.

LIVING WITH LACK

The following list demonstrates what will be created if there is a lack of these components in the physical body:

Lack of:	Will Create:
First Plane: Minerals	Lack of support
Second Plane: Vitamins	Lack of love
Third Plane: Proteins	Lack of nurturing
Fourth Plane: Carbohydrates	Lack of energy
Fifth Plane: Lipids	Lack of spiritual balance
Sixth Plane: Nucleic acid	Lack of spiritual structure
Seventh Plane: ATP	Lack of spirit

The First Plane: If you have a lack of minerals in the body, you will have lack of support on an emotional level and will be prone to diseases that have to do with a lack of support, such as some kinds of arthritis.

The Second Plane: If you have a lack of vitamins, you will have a lack of love on some level. Conversely, if you have a lack of love, you will not absorb your vitamins correctly.

The Third Plane: If you have a lack of proteins, you will have a lack of nurturing.

The Fourth Plane: If you have a lack of carbohydrates, there will be a lack of energy.

The Fifth Plane: If you have a lack of lipids, you will be without balance in your system and your hormones will be off. Hormones keep your body balanced.

The Sixth Plane: If you have a lack of nucleic acid, you will have a lack of structure in your life.

The Seventh Plane: If you have a lack of ATP, you will have a lack of spirit in your life. ATP is an important substance for the body's metabolism. When it is broken down, it releases large amounts of energy that can be utilized by cells and tissues to perform their functions. It is sometimes called universal energy. It is the energy that makes the cells function, the *pure energy* that is held on the mitochondria. The mitochondria are the essence that we get from our mother's DNA. The spirit is in the mitochondria, not in the DNA. The DNA is the computer programme, the mitochondria are the conscious electricity. When people die and energy is seen leaving the body, this is the mitochondria beginning to leave the physical dimension. A lack of ATP and hence low spiritual energy may mean that we have too many soul fragments in too many places and need to replenish these spent energies.

THE POWER OF THOUGHT

Thoughts are real things. They have essence. They can create anything in the planes of existence. We know this for a fact, because when we staged an Intuitive Anatomy class in Hawaii, we cleared so many issues from the students that by the end of the three weeks, everyone was acid–alkaline balanced at 7.2 alkaline. Technically, you have to eat alkaline-based food to keep your alkalinity at 7.2, and then nothing can make you ill. But it's not usually a straightforward process. I know by experience that even when clients are given straight alkaline foods, they still stay acidic for months. They go through huge healing crises and other dramas while their body alkalizes. Yet belief work made my entire class 7.2 alkaline in a short period of time and they were still eating chocolate cake. Your beliefs can create exactly the same energy as a vitamin, mineral or nutrient.

Do you know that if people take the amino acid or vitamin that they are lacking for the period of a month they clear up many of their emotional and unconscious issues? Also, they may stabilize and then don't have to take the supplements anymore.

Do you also know that you are supposed to be able to handle all of life's issues? Like a fine-tuned machine, that's how you're designed. Do you know that you are designed to survive raising teenagers? It's true!

Do you know that when a nursing mother kisses her baby she intuitively makes the right nutrients for its next feed? As a baby, I was bottle fed. Also, when my mother was pregnant with me, she was so sick that I missed out on nutrients in the womb. Her gallbladder was so bad and she had so many infections that they were surprised she was even alive. She had to have surgery and when they cut her open, they found she was pregnant with me. The doctors told her that she would never carry me and that I would have to be aborted. Do you know what she said to me recently? 'Look into my eyes, Vianna, and bond with me. We never bonded when you were born because I never thought I would carry you.' It is sad that she carried those thoughts all those years. It was great to have an opportunity to clear those beliefs.

USING THE PLANES TO HEAL

THE EQUATIONS OF THE PLANES OF EXISTENCE

Healers should always use more than one plane of existence at a time. This is called an *equation*.

The healer plays an important role in this equation as the witness:

Creator + Person to Be Worked On + Witness = Result.

Anytime that you use any plane of existence, you are actually using two or more planes at once. Every time you are using First-Plane energy, you are automatically using the Sixth Plane with it, for example. This is useful because the minerals from the First Plane can interact with the Law of Electricity to become even more potent.

HEALING MODALITIES

All healing modalities have their own significance within the planes of existence. For instance, acupuncture uses the Sixth, Third, Second and First

Planes of Existence and it works wonders. ThetaHealing is not in competition with any other healing modality, *especially modern medicine*.

Everything that you have learned from every healing modality and from every religion you have ever studied has brought you to this point where you can say to yourself, 'I want to clear my issues fast' and 'I have the ability to do what I am here to do.' You have gained experience with all the modalities.

INITIATIONS OF THE PLANES

Once, every time an advance was made or mastership of a plane was attained, a person would undergo an initiation, a giant mental shift, and because of the drama held on all of the planes, this could be traumatic. In ThetaHealing, because we have learned not to be bound to the planes, we can free our minds and therefore advance less traumatically.

We advance nevertheless: whenever you go up to the Creator and ask for a healing or go up and ask for a blessing for the Earth, you open your mind-spirit to new possibilities and levels and go through initiations accordingly. Have you ever felt or heard a psychic voice tell you that you have gone through an initiation? Have you ever had a near-death experience? A near-death experience, or death door, can be a healer's initiation into the growth process of development. The 'little death', as it is called, is the psychic doorway to another plane of existence.

With the belief work, we are able to pass initiations smoothly without having to sacrifice or die for attainment. *In fact, the belief work is the initiation.*

ATTACHMENT TO INDIVIDUAL PLANES

While I do my best to connect to the Seventh Plane while doing healings, the person that I am in the session with may be only receptive to the energy of a certain plane. One way to tell if a person is held in a hidden belief system of the Fifth Plane, for instance, is when you see a high angel coming to assist in the healing. This indicates that the person has vows, commitments or connections to the Fifth Plane of Existence. If the angel is assisting in the healing and only the energy of the Fifth Plane is used, then the angel will only work on the person in layers, because that is all they are allowed to do.

Because we are so intertwined with all of the other planes, we sometimes keep commitments and obligations from them and don't go up to the Creator first. We become so used to only using certain planes that we become bound by their rules. If you go up and ask the Creator of All That Is to do something, however, the energy will combine the planes and work in a different equation.

Something to bear in mind also is that an old soul will have instinctual elements of power from the collective consciousness, as well as past-life or ancestral memories, and may have brought an intimate knowledge of a particular plane of existence with them to this space and time.

Let us say that a person's spirit knows the secrets of the Fourth Plane and the power of shamanistic energy from it. Along with that shamanic energy, the person has certain limitations that have been put in place by their own beliefs or by the beliefs of the spiritual energies employed by the adept who taught them or even by the consciousness of the human condition at that time. This is not to say that shamanism is or was not evolved, or that the consciousness of certain individuals was so, only to state that perhaps the person's abilities in that place and time were regulated by the dictates of that particular plane of existence and the limitations of the collective consciousness that they tapped into at that time. So they learned these past limitations well, perhaps *too* well, and have now brought them into the present space and time, as well as the belief that *there are limitations*. They are therefore affected by these rules and regulations in this place and time.

In another instance, a healer may be in a room with a person whose neck is hurting, when all of a sudden the healer's neck hurts and the other person's pain is gone. This, too, is shamanic and happens because of the obligations, vows and commitments that the healer has carried into this life from the last.

Remember, too, that a person may be attempting to recapture the remembered elements of power held in another place and time, only to be disappointed by the fact that some of these elements must be re-created through initiations in the present. The ascended master of the Fifth Plane, for example, is constantly reminded of the limitations of the human body and faced with the collective belief systems of other inhabitants of this existence. This is one of the initiations facing the old soul: that of reconstructing the elements of power in this life and not constantly pining for the past one.

SENDING OUT AND BRINGING IN

In a healing, you should always first go up and connect to the Creator, then go to the specific plane of existence that you have chosen to use whatever power is on that plane.

The knowledge and energy of the Seventh Plane will always give you the highest and best answer to the situation and will elevate you beyond the limitations of the Law of Cause and Effect. In this way, you are on a quest towards walking in harmony with all the planes of existence and attaining mastership.

If you want to use the energy of All That Is, you must of course have the correct consciousness to get to the Seventh Plane. I suggest calling on the

Creator of All That Is. This phrase, created as a living thought form, with the unequivocal knowledge that it is sent out of your space to the Seventh Plane, will get you to the correct energy.

When I suggest you to go to the Seventh Plane, I advise you to witness the 'dis-creation' the illness. This means that you must create the reality that there is no illness. Tell the body that it is denied and there is a new scenario. In order for you to do this, you have to clear up limiting beliefs that tell you that you can't create in this way.

When some people perform energy healing, they go up above their space and command the energy to come through their body and out through their hands. Even though this energy comes from the Seventh Plane, it goes all the way through the healer's body before going into the person being healed and it is possible that, since the healer is only semi-divine, it is changed in the process. It still comes out as healing energy, but it has been filtered through the Third-Plane beliefs of the healer. Because of this the healing may not work as well.

17

FREE-FLOATING MEMORIES

The exercises in the following chapters are a few of the processes that are taught in the Advanced ThetaHealing class.

✧✧✧✧✧

The exercise for free-floating memories was given in *ThetaHealing*, but is worth repeating here. It was inspired by a woman who called me with her concerns about the seizures she was having. She wanted to have a baby and couldn't get pregnant because the seizure medication she was using would cause birth defects. When I was giving her a reading, I asked the Creator what could be done to stop her seizures. I was given the direct answer: *'Vianna, pull all of her free-floating memories.'*

I understood a little about free-floating memories from some things my ex-husband had taught me years before. They are recordings in the brain that have been imprinted by events, traumatic or otherwise, that have taken place at some point when we have been unconscious, whether through surgery, accidents, wartime trauma, extreme abuse or excessive alcohol or drug use.

Do you know that your brain is always conscious? Even when you are asleep, you are aware of everything that is happening in your life. When you are unconscious, you are still able to hear what is going on around you. Think of all the people who have had surgery or been knocked unconscious – all the words that have been said at that time have been recorded in their brain. This can be highly significant if you are having surgery on a cancerous tumour, or even on a non-cancerous tumour when the doctor says something like 'I think it's cancerous.'

The point is that when the mind is *conscious*, it knows how to process events properly. When it is *unconscious*, it may not do so and events can become free-floating memories. These memories can replay over and over, because whenever the words, noise or situation that took place when the person was unconscious are repeated in the waking world, they will relive the trauma. So, if you have a client who seems resistant to healing, check for free-floating memories.

With my client, I did as the Creator instructed me: I witnessed all the free-floating memories that were not for her highest good being released from her brain. Apparently, a situation in the past while she was unconscious had caused her to begin having seizures. Every time she smelled, heard or experienced something that was similar to the original situation, a seizure was triggered.

Her husband called me the next day, telling me that she had had another seizure. I worked with her again and witnessed the same process. This time her seizures stopped for good.

After her sessions with me, the doctors were able to take her off her seizure medication and she had a child the following year. She came to one of my seminars in California and showed me her little baby.

It is possible that many of us have free-floating memories that are hindering us from developing to our full potential.

To release a free-floating memory using ThetaHealing, follow this process:

THE PROCESS FOR RELEASING FREE-FLOATING MEMORIES

1. Centre yourself in your heart and visualize going down into Mother Earth, which is a part of All That Is.

2. Visualize bringing up energy through your feet, opening each chakra to the crown chakra. In a beautiful ball of light, go out to the universe.

3. Go beyond the universe, past the white lights, past the dark light, past the white light, past the jelly-like substance that is the Laws, into a pearly iridescent white light, into the Seventh Plane of Existence.

4. Make the command: *'Creator of All That Is, it is commanded that any free-floating memory that is no longer needed, that no longer serves this person, be pulled, cancelled and sent to God's light, in the highest and best way, and be replaced with the Creator's love. Thank you! It is done. It is done. It is done.'*

5. Move your consciousness over to the client and witness the healing taking place. Watch as the old memories are sent to God's light and the new energy from the Creator of All That Is replaces the old.

6. As soon as the process is finished, rinse yourself off and put yourself back into your space. Go into the Earth, pull Earth energy up through all your chakras to your crown chakra and make an energy break.

This process is beneficial to those who have been ill for a period of time, those who have had operations or those who have heard a doctor say that they are terminally ill, particularly if they have heard negative things or experienced negative trauma while unconscious. The release of these free-floating memories permits the mind to create a new scenario of belief in health.

I use this exercise, along with the 'Sending Love to the Baby in the Womb' and 'Heal the Broken Soul' exercises (*see following chapters*), whenever I am working with someone who is terminally ill. I have found that these exercises should be used more than once. The brain will release as many free-floating memories as it possibly can at one time, but it may not release them all. If the person has had many operations, for example, this exercise may need to be done several times.

18

SENDING LOVE TO THE
BABY IN THE WOMB

Again, this exercise was presented in *ThetaHealing*, but is of such importance that it is worth including again here.

CONCEPTION

How were you conceived? Were you wanted or not? Some of you may have been born when people weren't using contraceptives as they are now. Was your mother happy when you were born or was she overwhelmed? What was your reception like?

It was the custom of the ancient Hawaiians never to say a bad word around a woman who was pregnant. It was thought that if you got in an argument with your spouse when she was pregnant, there would be punishment after the birth. Before Christians settled on the islands, the people believed that a baby needed to have the best chance of survival possible and it had to be born and raised surrounded by good energy and good vibrations.

What were your parents talking about when *you* were born? Was there excitement and welcome energy, or were they fighting? Where they pleased that you were coming? When you arrived, was it warm? Were you taken away from your mother? Were you breastfed? All these memories are kept inside your body. Every word that was said at that time has been absorbed. What words made you feel inadequate, not worthy, guilty, wonderful and proud of yourself?

From the moment you are conceived, you are aware of everything around you. Your mother's feelings and beliefs are often brought to you in the womb. You can feel her traumatic thoughts, feelings of not wanting a child, fears of being overwhelmed and other stresses, and they will affect your noradrenaline and serotonin levels. Alcohol and drugs also affect a fetus' mental health and physical development.

THE 'SENDING LOVE TO THE BABY IN THE WOMB' EXERCISE

This exercise is an amazing healing process. It can benefit many diseases, such as alcohol fetal syndrome, bipolar disorder, attention deficit disorder and autism, and may simply eliminate them altogether. It also seems to help with the psychological effects of epilepsy, asthma and other things that are related to the formation of the foetus in the womb.

Some babies start out as twins, but nature only allows about one-third of the twins that are conceived to be born. This sometimes causes severe loneliness in the remaining twin. This loneliness can follow a person throughout their life, but this exercise takes care of it. It also sends the energy of the other child to the light.

You can do this exercise on yourself, on your children and on your parents – realizing, of course, that they have free agency as to whether they accept it or not. It is one of the few exercises that you can do without the verbal acceptance of a family member. This is because those you are genetically connected to will either unconsciously accept or deny the healing that is being sent to them.

This exercise did amazing things to my relationship with my mother. It has helped fathers, mothers and their children come together after many years of arguments and dissension. I suggest you use it on your clients and on yourself. *With clients, you must have their verbal consent to do this exercise.*

THE PROCESS FOR SENDING LOVE TO THE BABY IN THE WOMB

1. Centre yourself in your heart and visualize going down into Mother Earth, which is a part of All That Is.

2. Visualize bringing up energy through your feet, opening each chakra to the crown chakra. In a beautiful ball of light, go out to the universe.

3. Go beyond the universe, past the white lights, past the dark light, past the white light, past the jelly-like substance that is the Laws, into a pearly iridescent white light, into the Seventh Plane of Existence.

4. Make the command: *'Creator of All That Is, it is commanded that love be sent to this person as a baby in the womb. Thank you! It is done. It is done. It is done.'*

5. Now go up and witness the Creator's unconditional love surrounding the baby, whether that baby is you, your child or your parents. Witness love filling the womb and enveloping the fetus and simply eliminating all poisons, toxins and negative emotions.

6. As soon as the process is finished, rinse yourself off and put yourself back into your space. Go into the Earth, pull Earth energy up through all your chakras to your crown chakra and make an energy break.

19

HEALING THE BROKEN SOUL

Much of the information that I am given comes when I am doing classes. The 'Healing the Broken Soul' process came in when I was teaching the first Intuitive Anatomy class in Australia. One of the students was completely devastated by the loss of her daughter. She was so overwhelmed that she could not recover from it. She was sad and despondent in class and no matter how much belief work I did with her, she kept repeating the pitiful words, 'I am broken.'

That night I asked the Creator how I could help her and I heard, *'Vianna, heal her broken soul. She has a broken soul from all the sadness in her life.'*

I asked the Creator if *I* had a broken soul and I heard, *'Absolutely.'*

I said, 'But I've been pulling back my soul fragments all this time! I can't possibly have a broken soul.'

Then I was shown in my mind's eye what I can only describe as a crack in the bubble of energy that comprised my soul. I asked the Creator to heal my broken soul and I witnessed the crack being healed and my soul beginning to be reborn. I saw old hurts that I had never released, old sorrows and pain that I had been just too busy to mourn, being healed.

I was surprised at what cleared. I was sure that it would be abuse, but apparently I had already dealt with that. What came up was completely unexpected.

Around the time my children's father and I first began to break up, I had a collision with another car that knocked me into someone's front yard. I used their telephone to call my husband to come and get me. I told him that I had wrecked the car and he told me that he would come and get me once the football game was over. There I was, hurt, scared and vulnerable, and he told me that he would finish watching his football game first! At that moment, I realized that I was not going to be able to raise my children in a normal situation with this person and it was *over*. It was the pain from this incident that cleared when the Creator healed my broken soul.

The next morning I felt very different. That day I did the same work with the woman in the class. I witnessed the Creator heal her broken soul and she felt much better, too. This is where the process comes from.

I realized that the soul can be broken by many kinds of strange and harsh events in this life. When someone's feelings are irreparably hurt or they don't have proper time to grieve, a fracture can form in the energy of the soul. This explained the pattern I had begun to notice in many of my clients with cancer. You could fill them to the brim with all kinds of energy, but they just couldn't hold it. The healings would just *disappear* into them. Now I know that this was because their soul was broken.

Soon after this process was shown to me, I went to teach one of the early Advanced classes in Seattle, Washington. Some of my Intuitive Anatomy students were attending and I did the broken soul work with them. They all did very well except for one person, who had a hard time with it. She had been a bit of a challenge prior to this and I suspect that she had some competition issues with me. I have rarely felt such anger and jealousy from a student. During the process, because it took a little time for her soul to come back together, she decided to go up out of her space and cancel the process. This left her unfinished on almost every level and she began to act in a very unstable manner. She became unbalanced that night and caused quite a drama with her fellow Intuitive Anatomy graduates. As time went on, fortunately she became more composed, thanks to the support of her classmates. Anytime that you are going to heal the broken soul of another person, it is best to be sure that they are mentally stable.

I kept hoping that that particular student would get over her feelings towards me. However, to this day I do not think she has and, sad to say, I do not think she has overcome her aversion to the 'Healing the Broken Soul' exercise either. This is an example of why it is so important for the practitioner to see the process *finished* and for the client to permit them to do so.

After that fiasco, I was a little leery about teaching the technique. Nevertheless, when the next Advanced DNA class in Idaho Falls came up, God said, 'You are going to teach them how to heal their broken souls today.' More details followed:

*'Vianna, you are not putting together multiple personality disorders. You are not healing their broken **brain**, but healing parts of their **soul**. You must never leave before the process is finished. You must witness it until the spinning ball that represents their soul spins clockwise. If you leave them with the energy going counter-clockwise, it will bring up all their old issues from the past and they will have to deal with them before they can allow their soul to heal. This will leave them in a dilemma for a couple of days. If you finish it completely, they will be fine.'*

So I went ahead and taught the technique. However, some of the people were a little afraid of the process and they 'decorated' it too much, instead of just witnessing the Creator do the work. This made them go through trauma. Because of their interference in the work, what could have been done in 30 seconds took them three days to finish.

The Law of Truth had told me that when someone died, their soul went to the Creator and, through the Creator, was repaired. Now the Law of Truth gave me this alternative (truth always gives us alternatives): '*Vianna, heal the soul and the rest will follow.*'

I asked, 'If this is true, then why did you teach me to heal the body before the soul?'

I heard: 'Vianna, you were taught according to your needs. You had to be taught how to heal the body then heal the mind before you could learn to heal the soul. This was because you were not ready. This was what your mind could accept at the time, and you had to be clear about one thing at a time.'

It was true – I had first learned to heal the physical body while in a deep Theta brainwave. Then I had realized that the mind could interfere with the healing, so I had been given the belief work. Only then had I been taught that the soul might need to be healed as well.

HEALING THE BROKEN SOUL

The soul is magnificent! People don't realize that it is more divine and expansive than the body. Our souls are so expansive that we can be in more than one place dimensionally and more than one place in time.

For every lifetime there is a cord attached to our soul. This is connected to all the planes of existence. I believe that we are part of all the planes at once. And our energy is incredible. As part of the Creator, we are perfect in our own way.

But, just as we have a human body that can be broken, we sometimes accumulate emotional issues to the extent that cracks begin to form in the energy field of the soul. Sometimes life can become so intense in this illusion of reality that we become overwhelmed by the harshness of this existence and all the terrible things that have happened to us. Because of this despondency, we may feel empty to the very core of our being. This is the *grief that is beyond grief.*

Extreme physical and emotional illnesses can also break the spirit, causing damage to the soul. The spirit is different from the soul. The *spirit* is inside our body. The *soul* is everything we are.

If our energy becomes too fractured, we will die in order to make the repairs to our soul. In the greater awareness, this is a small matter and an accepted mode of repair to the soul. To the soul, death is not a big deal. Here on the Third Plane, we have this truly unusual concept of death: we always act as though it's the end. But really, it's just another step.

So, the old way to heal the soul was for it to leave this place, but now there is another process. Some people will still rather die to heal their soul because it has become so broken, but the 'Healing the Broken Soul' process can help them, too.

When you are working with someone, you should first ask the Creator of All That Is if their soul has been broken. Do not use energy testing, as it will not be accurate on this particular challenge. Go into the person's space and if they have a broken soul, you will see a ball of energy that has cracks and or tears in it.

When someone says, 'I'm so broken,' this is also an indication that you need to heal the broken soul.

I suggest that you work with a person on their belief systems first, so they will trust you and allow you to heal their soul. Trust is very important in any healing.

You should also ask the Creator of All That Is what to do for the person spiritually, as the healing criteria will not be the same from one person to the next.

One truth is apparent: a broken soul cannot be repaired but must be *re-created*. When the Creator of All That Is does this, the individual will become stronger as a result of the experience. As the phoenix rises from the ashes of death, so there is rebirth; through rebirth, there is creation.

THE PROCESS FOR HEALING THE BROKEN SOUL

First I want you to look into the person's eyes because the eyes are the windows to the soul. You have taken these eyes with you in every lifetime. This means that even in the spirit world your eyes have been the same.

1. Centre yourself.

2. Begin by sending your consciousness down into the centre of Mother Earth, which is a part of All That Is.

3. Bring the energy up through your feet, into your body and up through all your chakras.

4. Go up through your crown chakra in a beautiful ball of light, out past the stars to the universe.

5. Go beyond the universe, past the white lights, past the dark light, past

the white light, past the jelly-like substance that is the Laws, into a pearly iridescent white light, into the Seventh Plane of Existence.

6. Gather unconditional love and make the command: *'Creator of All That Is, it is commanded that* [name the person]*'s broken soul be healed and made whole once again at this time. Thank you! It is done. It is done. It is done.'*

7. Move your conscious into the person's crown chakra and go up and witness the healing. You may see a ball of light, or an orb, with cracks or tears in it. Watch as the Creator causes the ball to spin counter-clockwise then slow down to a full stop. Then watch as the sphere begins to spin clockwise and the cracks and tears become whole. Occasionally, you may just be out in the universe, but wait until the ball appears. Never question what you witness; that's not your job. Your job is just to witness. Some people may take longer than others. If the person you're working on appears despondent, go back and ask the Creator if their process has finished. Avoid cancelling the technique in the middle. As with all healing, wait until it seems finished and ask, 'Creator, is it finished?' Then wait for the answer.

8. When it is finished, connect back to the energy of All That Is, take a deep breath in and make an energy break if you so choose.

When you are witnessing the soul being healed, the first thing that you may see is it starting to turn clockwise, then counter-clockwise. It may open up like a lotus flower. You may see the spiritual energies of drug addictions flying off from it and there may be archetypical symbols. If you see energies flying back in from the outside, these are likely to be soul fragments. When we pull back our soul fragments, additional energy is added to the soul.

As the soul is healing, the energy will turn to the physical body of the person. It will come down into the heart chakra and spin around, and then you will see it turn into a giant sphere of light. The process isn't complete until you see this sphere turn clockwise. If you leave without witnessing this, the person will be processing emotions for hours, days, weeks or even months. Sometimes the healing process takes a considerable time, so be patient. The longest one that I have witnessed took 15 minutes.

Once the broken soul is healed, the person is going to have energy that they haven't had for a while. The process puts energy back into the mitochondria and infuses ATP back into the cells. When the soul is repaired, it will be possible to find and heal programmes and physical ailments that were difficult to see before.

The soul is like the Axis Mundi, the World Tree. The Creator is the whole tree, the Earth and everything else. The big branch is the soul, the little branch is the higher self and the leaf is the body.

20

THE HEART SONG

In July 2006, I began to feel extremely fatigued. Thinking that it was my lungs that were the problem, I began to do healings on them. While I was in the process of one of these healings, the voice of the Creator came into my head and asked, 'What are you doing?'

I replied, 'I am working on my lungs.'

The Creator said, 'It's not your lungs. You have congestive heart failure.'

In utter despair I cried, 'That's impossible! I am too young.'

To confirm that this is what I had, I made an appointment with the doctor. After putting me through some tests, the doctor said, 'You have congestive heart failure. I am so sorry.'

I asked, 'What am I supposed to do about it? How is it healed?'

The doctor said, 'Try this medicine and see if it works. Since you are young, we can put your name on a waiting list for a heart transplant.'

In this moment of desolation I cried to myself, 'Not again! Once again a doctor is telling me that I am going to die.' I went into the 'poor me' abyss. What really upset me about the whole situation was that I had done so much belief work and now I knew I had to do more.

I started taking the medicine, thinking, 'Well, I've promised to go and do the next ThetaHealing seminar. I must keep my promise.'

About two weeks before I left for Rome, where I was due to do the seminar, I had some guests over to my house. They were professional musicians from New York who were taking my Intuitive Anatomy class. They had come to have dinner and play some music. One of them played a magnificent viola and the sound that came from this instrument was full of melancholy and pulled at your heartstrings.

Then the other musician asked me to help him to compose some music with him. They told me to sing the music I had in my heart. I went up and connected to the Seventh Plane and began to sing in a mournful tone, feeling a strange emotion coming from my heart. As I felt these energies being lifted from me through the tone I was singing, I suddenly saw all the reasons for my unhappiness and the reasons for my sickness. I realized that I was holding old sorrows in the molecules of my heart. I had always worked on my beliefs without thinking of setting my heart free from the ancient pains it was holding on to. That was why I had continued to feel a sort of unmovable sufferance in my heart. I closed my eyes and let all this sadness come out in a tone that came from my heart. I continued to hold this tone until I was out of breath and then I started over again.

When I had finished and the music stopped, I opened my eyes and saw that the people in the room were crying. At that moment, I realized that I had found a way for others to melt the pain and the suffering in their hearts too.

When we are born onto this planet, we all absorb some of its vibrations of sorrow, particularly those of us who are intuitive. Many healers know that there is always something lying in their hearts, a sad, melancholy feeling. When we go to the Seventh Plane and listen to the melody in our hearts, we immediately feel lifted up because we manage to melt the pain of the generations that preceded us. I have found that the best way to let the sadness go is a low tone, almost a murmuring. Shouting will not have the same effect.

What I didn't know at the time of this first heart song was that this process had healed my heart. I now use it in my Advanced classes to clear people of their sorrow.

THE TONE FROM THE HEART: THE HEART SONG

This exercise is designed to release sorrow and anger from the past and the present with a tone that comes from the heart, released in a continuous song. Each organ has its own song and we can release negative influences from each by singing this sad song.

To do this we must go up out of our space and make the command that sorrow is released from our heart, as outlined below. Only we are able to release the sorrow and pain in our own heart – no one else can do it for us. A practitioner cannot release it for a client; they can only assist the client by encouraging them to create the tone.

This process is directly connected to the collective consciousness of humanity. When this process is done we release the suffering of all of humanity on a universal level. Many of us who do this exercise will connect to the universal tone that releases anger, hatred and sorrow on a world level.

Remember that there are three molecules that are held in the body that go with the soul everywhere it goes: one in the pineal gland that releases emotions and physical programmes, one in the heart that releases old sorrow and anger, and one at the base of the spine. This process activates the molecule in the heart. The practitioner should guide the client through it in the following way:

THE PROCESS FOR THE HEART SONG

1. Centre yourself in your heart and visualize going down into Mother Earth, which is part of All That Is.

2. Visualize bringing up the energy through your feet, opening each chakra to the crown chakra. In a beautiful ball of light, go out to the universe.

3. Go beyond the universe, past the white lights, past the dark light, past the white light, past the jelly-like substance that is the Laws, into a pearly iridescent white light, into the Seventh Plane of Existence.

4. Make the command: *'Creator of All That Is, I command that sorrow be released from the song of the heart through a tone of my voice. Thank you. It is done. It is done. It is done.'*

5. Imagine going to the Law of Music and asking for the tone that will release the sorrow and anger from the heart. Imagine that you are going down deep into your heart. Listen to the sad song your heart sings. Let it come out in your voice, in the tone that you sing.

6. As you listen to the sound that the heart sings, listen to all the resentments, all the frustrations with war, famine, hatred and anger that are locked in the heart. Let the sound that is locked in the heart come out of your mouth and be released. Then do the same for all the organs in the body.

7. When you have finished, connect back to the energy of All That Is, take a deep breath in and make an energy break if you so choose.

Some pointers:

- The practitioner should encourage the client to let the tone come out of their mouth and to continue until all the negative aspects are released from the heart.

- The way to tell that the process has finished is that the client feels finished. They will feel as though they have released all the built-up sorrow and anger from the heart.

- This process may be done more than once if the client needs to release layers from the heart.

- The client may not completely trust releasing all the stored sorrow with another person. However, they can use the process when they are alone.

- The song sung from the heart is not loud, but a steady neutral tone.

A HEART SONG SESSION

Here is an example that took place in class:

Vianna to man: 'Go up and connect to the Creator and then come down to your heart. I want you to listen to its music, which is only lightly audible under the heartbeat. I want you to sing the melody you hear.'

The man begins to sing in a melancholy tone.

Vianna: 'You are setting this old energy free. How do you feel?'

Man: 'It feels as though something's opening up.'

Vianna: 'I'll teach you what it feels like to know that you are safe and you can make a difference. These concepts are connected to your heart. Do you accept these feelings?'

Man: 'Yes.'

He sings for 15 minutes and then seems finished.

Vianna: 'OK, I think you are done. How do you feel now?'

Man: 'I feel revived!'

Vianna: 'Are you exaggerating?'

Man: 'No, I am speaking from my heart!'

Vianna: 'How do you feel from an energetic point of view?'

Man: 'I feel I'm alive.'

Vianna to class: 'As you are doing this, touch the person's heart with your hand. How long have you felt this way in your heart?'

Man: 'I've always felt this sorrow, but now I feel free. It has been hard all this time, holding this sorrow. I've worked 15 minutes on it with you and I never knew such weird sounds could come out of my mouth. Somehow, I recognized them, though, and I saw my past lives from beyond the universe.'

Vianna to class: 'We are all different and this exercise can last either two or ten minutes, depending on the person. The first thing you should do with a client using this technique is to be patient and help the person maintain the tone until they have completely finished. Then you can teach the feeling that they are safe and have a place in this world.

'If the tone that you hear them singing is a happy tune, tell them to dig more deeply into their heart.

'My mother tried to do this exercise, but the music that came out made her feel too sad and she decided not to do it anymore. My younger daughter tried it and the only thing that she could sing was happy music. I think that reflected what was actually in her heart.'

Downloads for the Heart Song

'Everything I have experienced matters.'

'This time I know how to wake people up to their potential.'

21

CLEARING AND BELIEF WORK ON NON-ORGANIC MATERIAL

As you know, objects can hold memories, emotions and feelings, ghost imprints of everything that has gone on around them as well as inside them.

For this reason you can actually teach your house what it feels like to be a home. Take a good look at your home to see if you need to do belief work on it. If the house is old and has a lot of history in it, it can have residual energy from the people who have lived in it. Pull any curses that you find on the house and send any waywards to the light. Your home needs to resonate with soul and energy.

Teach your house what it feels like to have joy and compassion and it will heal the people who come into it and who live there.

If you are not comfortable in your home, make it so. Send any memories that have sorrow or sadness to God's light.

Use fountains and decorate with mirrors, since your home is a reflection of you. Get rid of any possessions that you don't like, including clothes. Decorate your world the way you want it to be. Since non-organic material collects thoughts and feelings, download it with those that you want it to have.

With belief work, you can also pull curses off of a piece of land and return soul fragments to it, just as you would with a person.

This exercise has also been given in *ThetaHealing*, but is worth repeating here. It is for instilling objects with beliefs and feelings that will reflect back to you the environment you wish to create. Variations of it can be used with any object.

1. Centre yourself.

2. Begin by sending your consciousness down into the centre of Mother Earth, which is a part of All That Is.

3. Bring the energy up through your feet, into your body and up through all the chakras.

4. Go up through your crown chakra, raise and project your consciousness out past the stars to the universe.

5. Go beyond the universe, past the white lights, past the dark light, past the white light, past the jelly-like substance that is the Laws, into a pearly irides-cent white light, into the Seventh Plane of Existence.

6. Gather unconditional love and make the command: *'Creator of All That Is, it is commanded to teach this object the feeling of [whatever you want to teach the object], in the highest and best way. Thank you. It is done. It is done. It is done.'*

7. Witness the healing.

8. When you have finished, connect back to the energy of All That Is, take a deep breath in and make an energy break if you so choose.

22

BENDING TIME

Ancient Greek riddle: What is it that swallows what is before it and what is behind it as well anyone who is watching?

Answer: Time. It devours the past and the future, as well as all observers.

In the co-creative process of ThetaHealing, time does not exist. It slows to a crawl or stops completely during the period when healing is being done through the Creator of All That Is. This occurs so that the incredible amount of work that is happening has time to finish without causing the client any difficulties on the physical, mental or spiritual levels. You must realize that once the command has been made and your mind has witnessed and accepted the healing, it has already been accomplished outside the present time and reality. Being the witness brings the healing into *this* aspect of time and reality. You must witness it being accomplished for it to truly materialize in the physical world. Witnessing an instant healing is an example of bending time.

Time is an illusion, a Law of Gravity and one of the friendlier Laws to bend. I found this out one day when I was driving to work and was late. I went above my space to visualize a clock. Watching the clock, I commanded to see myself going faster than the clock. So when I got to work I had to visualize time changing back! One can get nine hours of sleep in minutes this way. *This must be accepted*, however, or you may still feel tired!

The ability to bend the Law of Time to change events in a conscious sense is learned through the following process:

THE PROCESS FOR TIME

1. Centre yourself in your heart and visualize yourself going down into the Mother Earth, which is part of All That Is.

2. Visualize bringing up the Earth energy through your feet, opening up all of your chakras as you go. Go up out of your crown chakra, in a beautiful ball of light, out to the universe.

3. Go beyond the universe, past the white lights, past the dark light, past the white light, past the jelly-like substance that is the Laws, into a pearly iridescent white light, into the Seventh Plane of Existence.

4. Make the command, *'Creator of All That Is, it is commanded that time be changed through the Law of Time from the Sixth Plane of Existence [state changes] on this month, day, year, time. Thank you. It is done. It is done. It is done.'*

5. Go to the Sixth Plane of Existence and connect with the Law of Time, witnessing the Law making the desired changes.

6. When you have finished, connect back to the energy of All That Is, take a deep breath in and make an energy break if you so choose.

When you are able to do this exercise, this is a good sign that you are ready for DNA 3.

23

REMEMBER YOUR FUTURE

There is an old wives' tale that an intuitive can't see their own future. This is an untruth. Not only can they see their future, but they can create it as well.

In the mechanistic view of reality, you can't see your future, because it simply hasn't happened yet. I believe that past, present and future are the same thing, however, and that one does not exist independently of the others. I believe that we live in all three at once, and just as we can remember our past, we can also remember the future. I think that there is a part of our consciousness that is beyond the past, the present and the future, and this is the God-Self, the spark of creation that is within all of us and able to change reality.

If you connect to the Creator of the Seventh Plane and ask to *remember* your future, you can see it crystal clear. This takes practice. In many instances, the intuitive tries to make the future what they want, without considering others around them and their divine timing (*see following chapter*). But a good intuitive easily realizes that they are creating everything in their life and, in so doing, becomes aware of the lives and rights of others.

There are several ways to remember your future. One way is to go up to the Creator and ask to be taken by the Law of Time to the Akashic Records. I prefer to go up to the Creator of All That Is and stand at the edge of the universe, where you can see your past, present and future at the same time. This has the added advantage that once you connect to the Seventh Plane, if you don't like the future you see you can simply change it ... or better yet, just create it.

THE PROCESS FOR REMEMBERING YOUR FUTURE

1. Imagine going up to the Seventh Plane.

2. Make the command: *'Creator of All That Is, it is commanded that I see and remember my future now. Thank you. It is done. It is done. It is done.'*

With regard to your future, another thing to remember is that because the genetic lineage is a chain connecting the past with the present and the present with the future, the changing of programmes within us now will affect both our ancestors in the past and our relatives in the present, thus setting up changes for the future.

24

DIVINE TIMING

What do I mean by 'diving timing'?

- I believe that we exist on this plane in divinity and are divinely directed.

- I believe that some things are pre-planned and that we do them in this world because we want to do them.

- I believe that we belong to a soul family.

- I believe that as we develop, we come together with our soul families with divine timing.

- I believe that part of our divine truth is coming together and working on our belief systems.

- I believe that we are here to connect to the Creator's energy of All That Is and *to learn*. This is the really important thing: to learn something wonderful from this existence.

Each person has their own divine timing. This is given by the Creator in relation to the timing of all the other people on the Third Plane of Existence. It must be respected by all of us for our own sake. As tiny sparks of God, we have free agency, however, and in egotism and stubbornness there are times when we go against the flow of the timing of divinity. Then we wonder why things do not 'go our way'.

On a macrocosmic scale, the Earth itself has its own divine timing. This is why it is best to command to know what the divine timing of the Earth is on a grand scale. Once you have an awareness of this grand dimension of divinity, it will open up a new understanding that can be used in readings, healings and manifesting what you want in your life. When you understand the grand scheme of things, you will know when to manifest, what to manifest and, with this knowledge, how to manifest.

Divine timing will also give you a better understanding of what is going on when you're doing a reading or healing on a person. In some instances, it is useful to ask what their divine timing is.

Remember that divine timing is what has been planned. It is always for our highest good, even if we do not understand it. Belief work will help us to know and work with our own divine timing.

You may ask, 'Is it possible to change my divine timing?' Changing some things may be possible, but divine timing is a part of why we are here and what we have come here to do, so to change it is to go against this. For instance, the drive that I have to teach has to do with my own divine timing. Don't get me wrong – the future can always be improved upon if you can see it coming. But divine timing has to do with major events in your life and some of these cannot be changed. Some of these are babies and soulmates.

As an exercise in divine timing, connect to the Creator of All That Is and ask to see and know your *divine timing*. This is not the same as knowing your future, as outlined earlier. If you can accurately see your future and your divine timing, this is a sign that you are ready for DNA 3. Keep in mind this takes practice.

Instill within yourself these downloads:

'I know what divine timing is on all levels.'

'I know how to plan for the future.'

'I know what an opportunity is.'

'I know how to take advantage of an opportunity.'

'I know what it feels like to follow through.'

'I know what it feels like to plan for the future.'

'I know how to see the future.'

INITIATIONS AND DEATH DOORS

You will find that as you progress intuitively, the Creator of All That Is may tell you that you are going through a 'little initiation'. This means that you are progressing nicely and are now being given the opportunity to take the next step in your evolution. It is up to you, using free will, whether to accept or decline this ascension. Too often, we are resistant to change and make things complicated. If the initiation is accepted with grace, it will be an easy process. Pull the programme 'Initiations are difficult', for truly they are just markers on our progress as divine sparks of the Creator of All That Is.

'Death doors' are a form of initiation. They are simply there to tell you that you've accomplished all that you came to do and to offer you the choice to go to another plane. If you choose to stay, you will be given another objective to follow. Just because you have a death door opportunity doesn't usually mean that you have to take it, though sometimes you do have no choice in the matter – the Creator is calling you home. We have hundreds of death doors in our lifetimes, however, and aren't conscious of most of them. The choices are given to the higher self and, from there, to the soul.

When a person declines a death door, their life changes and they grow spiritually. With this transition, new guardian angels are appointed to them. This is an initiation of development.

To change any negative death door programmes, use the belief work. Energy-test the person and, with permission, pull and replace any programmes that are not for their highest good. Energy-test for 'I must have a death door to grow spiritually'. One replacement might be 'It is easy for me to learn and grow spiritually without drama'.

According to the Law of Free Will, you cannot go around and close people's death doors for them. Only they can choose to shut them. On a deep level, this choice is theirs to make. What you can do, however, is to teach them to use the belief and feeling work. If you teach them what it *feels like* to have a happy and joyful life, then they'll want to live. For instance, when you work with a woman with breast cancer, start by giving her these beliefs and feelings and her body will start to heal:

'It's OK to be happy.'

'It's OK to live.'

'I'm important.'

'I'm cherished.'

'I'm heard.'

'I'm listened to.'

'I can communicate.'

Always remember, though, that death is only another beginning.

NEAR-DEATH EXPERIENCES

A near-death experience is usually an initiation of growth. The trick is to go beyond the need to have a near-death experience in order to move up spiritually.

Most people have to go through some kind of initiation to grow. Initiations are usually directly connected to our divine timing. Each brings a deepening relationship with the Creator of All That Is and a transformation of our soul energy. It is important that we permit these transformations to happen. They do not need to be painful. Open your heart and say, 'Creator of All That Is, I'm ready for the next step.' Visualize the new energy coming in from the Creator, being instillled throughout the body on the four belief levels and being sent out into the All That Is of your soul-field. This process will permit you to go through an initiation in a few minutes instead of a few months.

With regard to initiations, however, watch out for the negative ego slipping into your life! When the ego is no longer your amigo, initiations can be *hard*.

Also, do not attempt to force the issue. You will ascend when you are ready. We each have our own divine timing and you will move up when the time is right. When you go up to the Creator of All That Is, see correctly and accept what you see, you are partway there.

25

BELIEFS, DOWNLOADS AND FEELINGS

The following downloads and feelings are some of those that I have found to be of benefit from belief work sessions of the past nine years. I suggest downloading these feelings if they apply.

Abilities

'I understand the Creator's definition of developing my abilities.'

'I understand what it feels like to use my abilities in the highest and best way.'

'I know how to live my daily life utilizing my abilities to the fullest.'

'I know the Creator's perspective on my abilities.'

'I know it is possible to realize the full potential of my abilities.'

Absorption

'I understand the Creator's definition of absorbing the life force.'

'I understand the Creator's definition of absorbing information.'

'I understand what it feels like to absorb information.'

'I know what information to absorb.'

'I know how to absorb information in the highest and best way.'

'I know how to live my daily life absorbing information.'

'I know it is possible to absorb information.'

Accomplishment

'I understand the Creator's definition of accomplishment.'

'I understand what it feels like to accomplish my goals in the highest and best way.'

Accuracy

'I understand the Creator's definition of accuracy.'

'I understand what it feels like to be accurate.'

'I know how to be accurate in the highest and best way.'

'I know how to live my daily life accurately.'

'I know the Creator's perspective on accuracy.'

Achieving your Highest Potential

'I understand the Creator's definition of my highest potential.'

'I understand what it feels like to achieve my highest potential.'

'I know how to achieve my highest potential.'

'I know how to live my daily life achieving my highest potential.'

'I know the Creator's perspective on my highest potential.'

'I know it is possible to achieve my highest potential.'

Action

'I understand the Creator's definition of action.'

'I understand what it feels like to take action.'

'I know when to take action.'

'I know how to take action in the highest and best way.'

'I know how to live my daily life with action.'

'I know the Creator's perspective on the best action to take.'

'I know it is possible to take action.'

Addiction

'I understand what it feels like to live without addiction.'

'I know how to live without addiction.'

'I know how to live my daily life without addiction.'

'I know the Creator's perspective on living without addiction.'

'I know it is possible to live without addiction.'

Adequacy

'I understand the Creator's definition of adequacy.'

'I understand what it feels like to be adequate.'

'I know how to be adequate in the highest and best way.'

'I know it is possible to be adequate.'

Admiration

'I understand the Creator's definition of admiration.'

'I understand what it feels like to admire myself without conceit.'

'I know how to admire others in the highest and best way.'

'I know how to live my daily life in admiration of the world around me.'

'I know the Creator's perspective on admiration.'

Agony

'I understand what it feels like to live without agony.'

'I know how to live without agony.'

'I know how to live my daily life without agony.'

'I know the Creator's perspective on living without agony.'

'I know it is possible to live without agony.'

Alcoholism

'I understand what it feels like to live without being an alcoholic.'

'I know how to live without being an alcoholic.'

'I know how to live my daily life without being an alcoholic.'

'I know the Creator's perspective on life without alcohol.'

'I know it is possible to live without alcohol.'

'I can live without alcohol in the highest and best way.'

Angels

'I understand the Creator's definition of an angel of light.'

'I understand what it feels like to be angelic.'

'I know how to be angelic in the highest and best way.'

'I know how to live my daily life being angelic.'

'I know the Creator's perspective on being angelic.'

'I know it is possible to be angelic.'

Answers

'Answers come to me easily.'

'I understand the Creator's definition of having the answers to questions.'

'I understand what it feels like to receive answers through the Creator.'

'I know the answers.'

'I know when to have answers.'

'I know how to have the highest and best answers.'

'I know the Creator's perspective on answers.'

'I know it is possible to receive answers through the Creator.'

Anxiety

'I am free from anxiety.'

'I have a healthy outlook on life.'

'I am happy and others around me can't bring me down.'

'I never break down or give up.'

'Life is a rewarding challenge I enjoy.'

'Good will always win in my life.'

'My life is full of goodness and hope.'

'I am a responsible person and I believe in myself.'

'Others respect my strength.'

'My senses seek positive feelings.'

'I can bring my future into a bright opportunity.'

'Positive thinking controls my mind.'

'I am never afraid or alone.'

'I am at one with life, past, present and future.'

'I control my destiny.'

'I understand what it feels like to be free from anxiety.'

'I know how to live without anxiety.'

'I know how to live my daily life without anxiety.'

'I know it is possible to live without anxiety.'

'I understand the Creator's definition of enjoying life.'

'I understand what it feels like to enjoy life.'

'I know how to enjoy life.'

'I know it is possible to enjoy life.'

'I understand what it feels like to have control of my thoughts.'

'I know how to control my thoughts.'

'I know how to live my daily life in control of my thoughts.'

'I know it is possible to control my thoughts.'

'I understand the Creator's definition of goodness and hope.'

'I understand what it feels like to have goodness and hope.'

'I know the Creator's perspective on goodness and hope.'

'I know it is possible to have goodness and hope.'

'I understand what it feels like to believe in myself.'

'I know how to believe in myself.'

'I know how to live my daily life believing in myself.'

'I know the Creator's perspective on believing in myself.'

'I know it is possible to believe in myself.'

'I know how to separate the feelings of another person from my own.'

Apathy

'I understand the Creator's definition of living without apathy.'

'I understand what it feels like to live without apathy.'

'I know how to live without apathy in the highest and best way.'

'I know how to live my daily life to live without apathy.'

'I know the Creator's perspective on life without apathy.'

'I know it is possible to live without apathy.'

Appreciation

'I understand the Creator's definition of appreciation.'

'I am appreciated by others.'

'I understand what it feels like to appreciate others.'

'I know how to be appreciated in the highest and best way.'

'I know how to live my daily life appreciatively.'

'I know the Creator's perspective on appreciation.'

'I know it is possible to be appreciated.'

Attracting Wealth

'I know how to attract positive people and situations.'

'I understand the Creator's definition of attracting wealth.'

'I understand what it feels like to attract wealth.'

'I know how to attract wealth in the highest and best way.'

'I know how to live my daily life attracting wealth.'

'I know the Creator's perspective on attracting wealth.'

'I know it is possible to attract wealth.'

Being Abandoned

'I know how to live my life without being abandoned.'

'I understand what it feels like to live without being abandoned.'

Being Abrasive

'I understand what it feels like to live my life without being abrasive.'

Being Adorable

'I am adorable to others.'

'I understand the Creator's definition of being adorable.'

'I understand what it feels like to be adorable.'

'I know how to be adorable in the highest and best way.'

'I know the Creator's perspective on being adorable.'

'I know it is possible to be adorable.'

Being Attractive

'Others see me as attractive.'

'I see myself as attractive.'

'I understand the Creator's definition of being attractive.'

'I understand what it feels like to be attractive.'

'I know how to be attractive in the highest and best way.'

'I know the Creator's perspective on being attractive.'

'I know it is possible to be attractive.'

Being the Best You Can Be

'I understand the Creator's definition of being the best I can be.'

'I understand what it feels like to be the best I can be.'

'I know how to be the best I can be in the highest and best way.'

'I know how to live my daily life being the best I can be.'

'I know the Creator's perspective on being the best.'

'I know it is possible to be the best I can be.'

Being Capable

'I am a capable person.'

'I understand the Creator's definition of being capable.'

'I understand what it feels like to be capable.'

'I know how to be capable in the highest and best way.'

'I know how to live my daily life being capable.'

'I know the Creator's perspective on being capable.'

'I know it is possible to be capable.'

Being Clumsy

'I understand what it feels like to live without being clumsy.'

'I know how to live my daily life without being clumsy.'

'I know it is possible to live my daily life without being clumsy.'

Being Composed

'I am always composed.'

'I understand the Creator's definition of being composed.'

'I understand what it feels like to be composed.'

'I know when to be composed.'

'I know how to be composed in the highest and best way.'

'I know it is possible to be composed.'

Being Enchanted

'I understand the Creator's definition of being enchanted.'

'I understand what it feels like to be enchanted.'

'I know how to be enchanted in the highest and best way.'

'I know how to live my daily life enchanted with the world.'

'I know the Creator' perspective on being enchanted.'

'I know it is possible to be enchanted.'

Being Energetic

'I understand the Creator's definition of being energetic.'

'I understand what it feels like to be energetic.'

'I know when to be energetic and when to rest.'

'I know how to be energetic in the highest and best way.'

'I know how to live my daily life energetically.'

'I know the Creator's perspective on being energetic.'

Being Ethical

'I understand the Creator's definition of being ethical.'

'I understand what it feels like to be ethical.'

'I know how to be ethical in the highest and best way.'

'I know how to live my daily life ethically.'

'I know the Creator's perspective on being ethical.'

'I know it is possible to be ethical.'

Being a Genius

'I understand the Creator's definition of being a genius.'

'I understand what it feels like to be a genius.'

'I know how to be a genius in the highest and best way.'

'I know it is possible to be a genius.'

Being Gentle

'I understand the Creator's definition of being gentle.'

'I understand what it feels like to be gentle in the highest and best way.'

'I know when to be gentle but firm.'

'I know the Creator's perspective on being gentle.'

'I know it is possible to be gentle.'

Being Genuine

'I understand the Creator's definition of being genuine.'

'I understand what it feels like to be genuine in the highest and best way.'

'I know when to be genuine.'

'I know how to be genuine.'

'I know it is possible to be genuine.'

Being Grounded

'I understand the Creator's definition of being grounded.'

'I understand what it feels like to be grounded.'

'I know when to be grounded.'

'I know how to be grounded in the highest and best way.'

'I know the Creator's perspective on being grounded.'

'I know it is possible to be grounded.'

Being Present

'I understand the Creator's definition of being present.'

'I understand what it feels like to be present.'

'I know when to be present.'

'I know how to be present.'

'I know how to live my daily life being present.'

'I know the Creator's perspective on being present.'

'I know it is possible to be present.'

Being Respected

'I understand the Creator's definition of being respected by
my friends.'

'I understand what it feels like to be respected by my friends.'

'I know how to be respected by my friends.'

'I know it is possible to be respected by my friends.'

'I understand the Creator's definition of being respected by
my teachers.'

'I understand what it feels like to be respected by my teachers.'

'I know how to be respected by my teachers.'

'I know it is possible to be respected by my teachers.'

'I understand the Creator's definition of being respected by my class.'

'I understand what it feels like to be respected by my class.'

'I know how to be respected by my class.'

'I know it is possible to be respected by my class.'

Being a Scholar

'I understand the Creator's definition of being a scholar.'

'I understand what it feels like to become a scholar.'

'I know how to become a scholar.'

'I know it is possible to become a scholar.'

Being Sensible

'I understand the Creator's definition of being sensible.'

'I understand what it feels like to be sensible.'

'I know when to be sensible in the highest and best way.'

'I know how to be sensible.'

'I know the Creator's perspective on being sensible.'

'I know it is possible to be sensible.'

Believing in Yourself

'I believe in myself.'

'I am a positive person.'

'I am good-natured and others admire my confidence.'

'I have great strength of conviction.'

'Hopes and dreams make me feel good.'

'I create my own confidence because I am successful.'

'Every day, in every way, I grow more successful.'

'I assert myself clearly.'

'I make the right decisions because I trust myself.'

'Being confident makes me feel good.'

Brilliance

'I understand the Creator's definition of the brilliance of my soul.'

'I understand what it feels like to be brilliant.'

'I know how to be brilliant.'

'I know the Creator's perspective on brilliance.'

Business

    'I know what it feels like to have a business.'

    'I know how to have a business.'

    'I know it is possible to have a business.'

    'I know how to run my business in the highest and best way.'

Change without Resistance

    'I understand what it feels like to experience change in the highest and best way without resistance.'

    'I know when to experience change without resistance.'

    'I know how to experience change without resistance.'

    'I know it is possible to experience change without resistance.'

Collaboration

    'I understand the Creator's definition of collaboration.'

    'I understand what it feels like to collaborate with others.'

    'I know when to collaborate with others.'

    'I know how to collaborate with others.'

    'I know how to live my daily life collaborating.'

    'I know the Creator's perspective on collaboration.'

    'I know it is possible to collaborate.'

Communication

    'I communicate well with others.'

    'I understand the Creator's definition of communication.'

    'I understand what it feels like to communicate.'

    'I know how to communicate in the highest and best way.'

    'I know the Creator's perspective on communication.'

    'I know it is possible to communicate.'

Comprehension

'I comprehend concepts easily.'

'I understand what it feels like to comprehend.'

'I know how to comprehend in the highest and best way.'

'I know how to live my daily life comprehending.'

'I know the Creator's perspective on comprehending others.'

'I know it is possible to comprehend.'

Concern

'I can be concerned for others in the highest and best way.'

'I understand the Creator's definition of concern for others.'

'I understand what it feels like to have concern for others.'

'I know when to have concern.'

'I know how to have concern in the highest and best way.'

'I know the Creator's perspective on concern for others.'

'I know it is possible to have concern for others.'

Confusion

'I understand what it feels like to live without confusion.'

'I know how to live without confusion in the highest and best way.'

'I know how to live my daily life without confusion.'

'I know it is possible to live without confusion.'

Consideration

'I understand the Creator's definition of consideration for others.'

'I understand what it feels like to have consideration.'

'I know when to have consideration.'

'I know how to have consideration.'

'I know how to live my daily life with consideration.'

'I know the Creator's perspective on consideration.'

'I know it is possible to have consideration.'

Controlling Temper

'I understand what it feels like to control my temper.'

'I know when to control my temper.'

'I know how to control my temper.'

'I know how to live my daily life controlling my temper.'

'I know it is possible to control my temper.'

Co-ordination

'I am a co-ordinated person.'

'I understand the Creator's definition of co-ordination.'

'I understand what it feels like to be co-ordinated.'

'I know how to be co-ordinated in the highest and best way.'

'I know how to live my daily life co-ordinated with the Creator.'

'I know the Creator's perspective on being co-ordinated.'

'I know it is possible to be co-ordinated.'

Creativity

'I create beautiful things.'

'I think wonderful thoughts.'

'I dream wonderful dreams.'

'I am a creative person.'

'I have fascinating ideas.'

'Every day, in every way, I become more creative.'

'I am creative in every way.'

'I enjoy being creative.'

'I find creative solutions.'

'I see new visions of creativity.'

'I find new ways to do things.'

'I dream of fantastic things.'

'I go to sleep and wake up creative.'

'I understand the Creator's definition of creativity.'

'I understand what it feels like to be creative.'

'I know how to be creative.'

'I know the Creator's perspective on creativity.'

'I know it is possible to be creative.'

'I understand what to create.'

'I understand what it feels like to think wonderful thoughts.'

'I understand what it feels like to dream wonderful dreams.'

'I understand how to be a creative person.'

'I understand what it feels like to download fascinating ideas from the Creator of All That Is.'

'I understand how to download fascinating ideas from the Creator of All That Is.'

'I understand what it feels like to solve difficult problems with creative solutions.'

'I understand what it feels like to offer creative advice.'

'I understand what it feels like to have a created vision.'

'I understand what it feels like to be intelligent and bright.'

'I understand what it feels like to be creative on all levels of my being: physically, emotionally, mentally and spiritually.'

The Creator's Voice

'I understand the Creator's definition of the Creator's voice.'

'I understand what it feels like to hear the Creator's voice.'

'I know what the Creator's voice is.'

'I know how to hear the Creator's voice.'

Curiosity

'I understand the Creator's definition of curiosity.'

'I understand what it feels like to be curious.'

'I know when to be curious.'

'I know how to be curious in the highest and best way.'

'I know how to live my daily life curious about my surroundings.'

'I know the Creator's perspective on curiosity.'

Deceit

'I understand what it feels like to live without being deceived.'

'I know how to live my daily life without being deceived.'

'I know it is possible to live without being deceived.'

Dependability

'I understand the Creator's definition of dependability.'

'I understand what it feels like to be dependable.'

'I know how to be dependable in the highest and best way.'

'I know the Creator's perspective on dependability.'

'I know it is possible to be dependable.'

Dignity

'I understand the Creator's definition of dignity.'

'I understand what it feels like to have dignity.'

'I know when to have dignity.'

'I know how to live my daily life with dignity.'

'I know the Creator's perspective on dignity.'

'I know it is possible to have dignity.'

Discipline

'I understand the Creator's definition of being disciplined and achieving my goals.'

'I understand what it feels like to be disciplined and achieve my goals.'

'I know when to be disciplined and achieve my goals.'

'I know how to be disciplined and achieve my goals in the highest and best way.'

'I know how to live my daily life in a disciplined way and achieve my goals.'

'I know the Creator's perspective on being disciplined and achieving goals.'

'I know it is possible to have discipline and achieve my goals.'

Divinity

'I understand the Creator's definition of divinity.'

'I understand what it feels like to be divine.'

'I know how to be divine in the highest and best way.'

'I know how to live my daily life in divinity.'

'I know the Creator's perspective on being divine.'

'I know it is possible to be divine.'

Dreams

'I understand the Creator's definition of making my dreams come true.'

'I understand what it feels like to have my dreams come true.'

'I know my dreams will come true.'

'I know when to have my dreams come true.'

'I know how to have my dreams come true.'

'I know how to live my daily life watching my dreams come true.'

'I know the Creator's perspective on dreams coming true.'

'I know it is possible to have my dreams come true.'

'I am worthy of having my dreams come true.'

'I know it's safe to dream.'

'I know when I am living my dream.'

Elegance

'I understand the Creator's definition of elegance.'

'I understand what it feels like to be elegant.'

'I know when to be elegant.'

'I know how to be elegant.'

'I know how to live my daily life elegantly.'

'I know the Creator's perspective on elegance.'

'I know it is possible to be elegant.'

Eloquence

'I understand the Creator's definition of eloquence.'

'I understand what it feels like to be eloquent.'

'I know when to be eloquent.'

'I know how to be eloquent.'

'I know how to live my daily life eloquently.'

'I know the Creator's perspective on eloquence.'

'I know it is possible to be eloquent.'

Empowerment

'I understand what it feels like to trust and believe in myself.'

'I understand what it feels like to have people trust me and believe in me.'

'I understand what it feels like to be accountable for my actions.'

'I understand what it feels like to make good choices.'

'I understand what it feels like to make correct decisions for myself and those around me.'

'I understand what it feels like to learn from the challenges of life.'

'I understand what it feels like to be independent.'

'I understand what it feels like to look forward to tomorrow.'

'I understand what it feels like when my mind is keen and aware.'

'I understand what it feels like to be patient with myself.'

'I understand what it feels like to be trustworthy.'

'I understand what it feels like to have high principles.'

'I understand what it feels like to be responsible for my destiny.'

'I understand what it feels like to be successful.'

Everlastingness

'I understand the Creator's definition of my everlastingness.'

Excitement

'I understand what it feels like to be excited in the highest and best way.'

'I know when to be excited.'

'I know how to live my daily life excited by life.'

'I know the Creator's perspective on excitement.'

'I know it is possible to be excited.'

Existence

'I understand the Creator's definition of my existence.'

Expansion

'I understand the Creator's definition of expansion.'

'I understand what it feels like to expand on all levels.'

'I know when to expand.'

'I know how to expand in the highest and best way.'

'I know the Creator's perspective on spiritual and mental expansion.'

'I know it is possible to expand.'

Fairy Magic

'I understand what fairy magic feels like in the highest and best way.'

Faithfulness

'I understand the Creator's definition of faithfulness.'

'I understand what it feels like to be faithful to others and myself.'

'I know how to be faithful in the highest and best way.'

'I know the Creator's perspective on being faithful.'

'I know it is possible to be faithful.'

Fascination

'I understand the Creator's definition of being fascinated with life.'

'I understand what it feels like to be fascinated.'

'I know how to be fascinated in the highest and best way.'

'I know how to live my daily life fascinated with life.'

'I know the Creator's perspective on fascination.'

'I know it is possible to be fascinated.'

Freedom

'I understand the Creator's definition of freedom.'

'I understand what it feels like to be free.'

'I know how to be free in the highest and best way.'

'I know how to live my daily life in freedom.'

'I know the Creator's perspective on freedom.'

'I know it is possible to be free.'

Frequency

'I understand the Creator's definition of my frequency of vibration.'

The Future

'I understand the Creator's definition of the future.'

'I understand what it feels like to remember the future.'

'I know how to remember the future in the highest and best way.'

'I know the Creator's perspective on the future.'

'I know it is possible to remember the future.'

Generosity

'I understand the Creator's definition of generosity.'

'I understand what it feels like to be generous.'

'I know when to be generous.'

'I know how to be generous in the highest and best way.'

'I know how to live my daily life generously.'

'I know the Creator's perspective on generosity.'

'I know it is possible to be generous.'

Genetics

'I understand the Creator's definition of genetics.'

'I know the Creator's perspective on genetics.'

Goals

'I understand the Creator's definition of having goals.'

'I understand what it feels like to have goals.'

'I know when to have goals.'

'I know how to have goals.'

'I know the Creator's perspective on goals.'

'I know it is possible to have goals.'

Gratitude

'I understand the Creator's definition of gratitude.'

'I understand what it feels like to be grateful.'

'I know when to be grateful.'

'I know how to be grateful.'

'I know how to live my daily life in gratitude.'

'I know the Creator's perspective on gratitude.'

'I know it is possible to be grateful.'

Growth

'I understand the Creator's definition of growth.'

'I understand what it feels like to grow.'

'I know how to grow in the highest and best way.'

'I know how to live my daily life in growth.'

'I know the Creator's perspective on growth.'

'I know it is possible to grow.'

Guilt

'I am here now.'

'I am alive.'

'I see clearly now.'

'I feel good now.'

'I feel good being in my body.'

'I am free.'

'I deserve a good life.'

'I hear clearly now.'

'I forgive myself.'

'I breathe now.'

'I understand the Creator's definition of living without compulsive guilt.'

'I understand what it feels like to live without compulsive guilt.'

'I know how to live my daily life without compulsive guilt.'

Healer Issues

'I understand the Creator's definition of being responsible for my power.'

'I have good judgement about my abilities.'

'I know what it feels like to love.'

'I know how to be completely loved and accepted.'

'I know what it feels like to have my peers accept me.'

'I know how to bring the right peers to me.'

'I know what it feels like to know whom I can trust.'

'I know how to attract people to me who are trustworthy.'

'I know the Creator's definition of what a friend is.'

'I know how to draw friends to me that match my vibration.'

'I know what it feels like to have the Creator's abundance.'

'I know what to do with the Creator's abundance.'

'I know what it feels like to have money.'

Healing

'I am happy.'

'I am healthy.'

'I eat good food.'

'I like to exercise.'

'I relax.'

'The pain is gone.'

'I can do it.'

'I am strong.'

'I like myself.'

'All is well.'

'I am good.'

'My body is powerful.'

'I understand the Creator's definition of healing.'

'I understand what it feels like to heal others.'

'I understand what it feels like to heal myself.'

'I understand the Creator's definition of an instant healing.'

'I know when to heal others.'

'I know how to heal others and myself.'

'I know how to live my daily life regenerating.'

'I know the Creator's perspective on healing.'

'I know it is possible to heal others and myself.'

'I know how to heal through the Creator of All That Is.'

Holism

'I understand the Creator's definition of seeing life holistically.'

'I know how to live my daily life holistically.'

Hope

'I understand the Creator's definition of hope.'

'I understand what it feels like to have hope in the highest and best way.'

'I know how to have hope in the highest and best way.'

'I know how to live my daily life with hope.'

'I know the Creator's perspective on hope.'

'I know it is possible to have hope.'

Illusion

'I understand the Creator's definition of illusion.'

'I understand what it feels like to see the illusion of life.'

'I know how to see the illusion of life.'

'I know the Creator's perspective on illusion.'

The Immune System

'Every day, in every way, my immune system is strong and resilient.'

'I understand the Creator's definition of what an immune system should be.'

'I understand what it feels like to have a strong and healthy immune system.'

'I know how to have a strong immune system in the highest and best way.'

'I know how to live my daily life with a strong immune system.'

'I know the Creator's perspective on a strong and healthy immune system.'

'I know it is possible to have a strong and healthy immune system.'

Improvement

'Every day, in every way, I feel and see improvements in my life.'

'I understand the Creator's definition of improvement.'

'I understand what it feels like to improve.'

'I know how to improve in the highest and best way.'

'I know how to live my daily life improving.'

'I know the Creator's perspective on improvement.'

'I know it is possible to improve.'

Initiative

'I understand the Creator's definition of having initiative.'

'I understand what it feels like to have initiative.'

'I know how to have initiative.'

'I know how to live my daily life with true initiative.'

'I know the Creator's perspective on initiative.'

'I know it is possible to have initiative.'

'I know how to take the next spiritual steps.'

'I am aware of another's space.'

'I am conscious of another's space.'

'I know how to live my daily life without the fear of the unknown.'

'I know how to live my daily life without the fear of the nothing.'

Insight

'Every day, in every way, I have more insight.'

'I understand the Creator's definition of insight.'

'I understand what it feels like to have insight in the highest and best way. '

'I know how to have insight.'

'I know the Creator's perspective on insight.'

'I know it is possible to have insight.'

Intelligence

'Every day, in every way, I become more intelligent.'

'I understand the Creator's definition of intelligence.'

'I understand what it feels like to be intelligent.'

'I know how to be intelligent in the highest and best way.'

'I know how to live my daily life intelligently.'

'I know the Creator's perspective on intelligence.'

'I know it is possible to be intelligent.'

Interaction

'I understand the Creator's definition of interacting with all situations.'

'I understand what it feels like to interact.'

'I know when to interact in all situations.'

'I know how to interact in all situations.'

'I know how to live my daily life interacting in all situations.'

'I know it is possible to interact in all situations.'

Magnificence

'I understand the Creator's definition of magnificence.'

'I understand what it feels like to be magnificent.'

'I know how to be magnificent in the highest and best way.'

'I know how to live my daily life magnificently.'

'I know the Creator's perspective on magnificence.'

'I know it is possible to be magnificent.'

Manifesting

'I understand the Creator's definition of manifesting.'

'I understand what it feels like to manifest in the highest and best way.'

'I know when to manifest.'

'I know how to manifest.'

'I know how to live my daily life manifesting good things.'

'I know the Creator's perspective on manifesting.'

'I know it is possible to manifest.'

Mastership

'I understand the Creator's definition of mastership.'

Memory

'I like myself.'

'My mind absorbs information like a sponge.'

'I can link thoughts together.'

'I have an infinite capacity to remember.'

'I remember vividly.'

'I remember pictures.'

'I recall events as they really happened.'

'I succeed in remembering faces, names and events.'

'I practise improving my memory daily.'

'I am relaxed and remember easily.'

'I recall information for tests easily.'

'I understand the Creator's definition of memory.'

'I understand what it feels like to have a good memory.'

'I know how to have a good memory. '

'I know it is possible to have a good memory.'

'I understand what it feels like to remember easily.'

'I know it is possible to have an infinite capacity to remember.'

'I understand what it feels like to remember in pictures.'

'I understand how to remember in pictures.'

'I understand what it feels like to associate the new with the old memories.'

'I understand what it feels like to remember in stressful situations.'

Mental Clarity

'I understand the Creator's definition of mental clarity.'

'I understand what it feels like to be mentally clear.'

'I know how to have mental clarity in the highest and best way.'

'I know how to live my daily life with mental clarity.'

'I know the Creator's perspective on mental clarity.'

'I know it is possible to have mental clarity.'

Mercy

'I understand the Creator's definition of having mercy.'

'I understand what it feels like to have mercy.'

'I know when to have mercy.'

'I know how to have mercy in the highest and best way.'

'I know how to live my daily life with mercy.'

'I know the Creator's perspective on having mercy.'

'I know it is possible to have mercy.'

Metaphysics

'I understand the Creator's definition of metaphysics.'

'I know how to be metaphysical in the highest and best way.'

'I know the Creator's perspective on metaphysics.'

'I know it is possible to be metaphysical without ego.'

Mysticism

'I understand the Creator's definition of mysticism.'

'I understand what it feels like to be mystical in the highest and best way.'

'I know when to be mystical.'

'I know how to be mystical.'

'I know the Creator's perspective on being mystical.'

'I know it is possible to be mystical.'

Nobility

'I understand the Creator's definition of nobility.'

'I understand what it feels like to be noble.'

'I know when to be noble.'

'I know how to be noble in the highest and best way.'

'I know how to live my daily life nobly.'

'I know the Creator's perspective on being noble.'

'I know it is possible to be noble.'

Omnipresence

'I understand the Creator's definition of omnipresence.'

'I understand what it feels like to be omnipresent with creation in the highest and best way.'

'I know how to be omnipresent with creation.'

'I know how to live my daily life being omnipresent.'

'I know the Creator's perspective on omnipresence.'

'I know it is possible to be omnipresent.'

Passion

'I understand the Creator's definition of passion.'

'I understand what it feels like to be passionate in the highest and best way.'

'I know when to be passionate.'

'I know how to be passionate.'

'I know how to live my daily life with passion.'

'I know the Creator's perspective on passion.'

'I know it is possible to be passionate.'

Patience

'I am a patient person.'

'Patience is tolerance.'

'Patience is understanding.'

'Patience is nature's way.'

'Patience is good.'

'I am patient with myself.'

'I am patient with others.'

'I enjoy being patient.'

'I understand the Creator's definition of patience.'

'I understand what it feels like to be patient.'

Possibilities

'I understand the Creator's definition of possibilities.'

'I understand what it feels like to have possibilities.'

'I know there are possibilities available to me.'

'I know when to have possibilities.'

'I know how to have possibilities in the highest and best way.'

'I know how to live my daily life with possibilities.'

'I know the Creator's perspective on possibilities.'

Potential

'I can grow in any direction.'

'I have limitless personal possibilities.'

'I am a positive person.'

'Each day marks a new peak in my personal awareness.'

'My spirit has no limit.'

'Independence is strength.'

'In my heart I have only goodness.'

'Others respect me and believe in my potential.'

'People know I am a strong person.'

Preciousness

'I understand the Creator's definition of life being precious.'

'I know the Creator's perspective on what is precious.'

Quietness

'I understand the Creator's definition of quietness.'

'I understand what it feels like to be quiet and listen to the Creator.'

'I know when to be quiet.'

'I know how to be quiet in the highest and best way.'

'I know the Creator's perspective on quietness.'

'I know it is possible to be quiet.'

Radiance

'I understand the Creator's definition of radiating joy to others.'

'I understand what it feels like to be radiant.'

'I know how to be radiant in the highest and best way.'

'I know how to live my daily life radiating positive rays.'

'I know the Creator's perspective on radiance.'

'I know it is possible to radiate the energy of the Creator of All That Is.'

Respecting Others

'I understand the Creator's definition of respecting another person.'

'I understand what it feels like to respect another person.'

'I know when to respect another person.'

'I know how to respect another person.'

'I know how to live my daily life respecting other people.'

'I know the Creator's perspective on respecting other people.'

'I know it is possible to respect other people.'

Rewards

'I understand the Creator's definition of rewards.'

'I understand what it feels like to be rewarded in the highest and best way.'

'I know when to reward others.'

'I know how to be rewarded.'

'I know the Creator's perspective on rewards.'

'I know it is possible to be rewarded.'

Rhythm

'I understand the Creator's definition of rhythm.'

'I know how to feel the rhythm of creation in the highest and best way.'

'I know how to live my daily life in rhythm.'

'I know the Creator's perspective on rhythm.'

'I know it is possible to have rhythm.'

Romance

> 'I understand the Creator's definition of romance.'

> 'I understand what it feels like to be romantic in the highest and best way.'

> 'I know when romance is for my highest good.'

> 'I know how to permit romance in my life.'

> 'I know the Creator's perspective on romance.'

> 'I know it is possible to be romantic with my partner.'

Satisfaction

> 'I understand the Creator's definition of satisfaction.'

> 'I understand what it feels like to be satisfied in the highest and best way.'

> 'I know when to be satisfied.'

> 'I know how to be satisfied.'

> 'I know how to live my daily life satisfied.'

> 'I know the Creator's perspective on satisfaction.'

> 'I know it is possible to be satisfied.'

Self-confidence

> 'I am self-confident.'

> 'People see me as self-confident.'

> 'I understand the Creator's definition of self-confidence.'

> 'I understand what it feels like to be self-confident.'

> 'I know how to be self-confident in the highest and best way.'

> 'I know how to live my daily life self-confidently.'

> 'I know the Creator's perspective on self-confidence.'

> 'I know it is possible to be self-confident.'

Self-control

'I understand the Creator's definition of self-control.'

'I know what self-control is.'

'I understand what it feels like to have self-control in the highest and best way.'

'I know when to have self-control.'

'I know how to have self-control.'

'I know how to live my daily life with self-control.'

'I know the Creator's perspective on self-control.'

'I know it is possible to have self-control.'

Significance

'I understand the Creator's definition of significance.'

'I understand what it feels like to be significant.'

'I know when to be significant.'

'I know how to be significant in the highest and best way.'

'I know how to live my daily life being significant.'

'I know the Creator's perspective on significance.'

'I know it is possible to be significant.'

Sincerity

'I understand the Creator's definition of sincerity.'

'I understand what it feels like to be sincere.'

'I know what sincerity is.'

'I know when to be sincere.'

'I know how to be sincere in the highest and best way.'

'I know how to live my daily life in sincerity.'

'I know the Creator's perspective on sincerity.'

'I know it is possible to be sincere.'

Smoking

'I can stop smoking.'

'I am smoking less until I quit smoking.'

'Smoking does not interest me.'

'I can break the habit of smoking.'

'I know what it feels like to stop smoking.'

'I know how to stop smoking.'

'I know how to live without smoking.'

'I know it is possible to live without smoking.'

Sophistication

'I understand the Creator's definition of sophistication.'

'I understand what it feels like to be sophisticated.'

'I know how to be sophisticated in the highest and best way.'

'I know how to live my daily life with sophistication.'

'I know the Creator's perspective on sophistication.'

'I know it is possible to be sophisticated.'

The Spark of Life

'I understand the Creator's definition of the spark of life.'

'I understand what it feels like to be a spark of the Creator of All That Is.'

Speaking and Writing

'I speak and communicate well.'

'Conversation comes easily to me.'

'I write interesting thoughts.'

'People are interested in my thoughts.'

'Words come naturally to me.'

'I am a spontaneous speaker.'

'I take complex thoughts and make them simple.'

'I speak and write my thoughts clearly.'

'I speak with ease and am easily understood.'

Spirituality

'I understand the Creator's definition of spirituality.'

'I understand what it feels like to be spiritual in the highest and best way.'

'I know the Creator's perspective on spirituality.'

'I know it is possible to be spiritual.'

Splendour

'I understand the Creator's definition of splendour.'

'I understand what splendour feels like.'

'I know the Creator's perspective on splendour.'

Spontaneity

'I understand the Creator's definition of spontaneity.'

'I understand what it feels like to be spontaneous.'

'I know when to be spontaneous.'

'I know how to be spontaneous in the highest and best way.'

'I know how to live my daily life in a spontaneous way.'

'I know the Creator's perspective on spontaneity.'

'I know it is possible to be spontaneous.'

Strength

'I understand the Creator's definition of strength.'

'I understand what it feels like to be strong.'

'I know what strength is.'

'I know how to be strong in the highest and best way.'

'I know how to live my daily life with strength.'

'I know the Creator's perspective on strength.'

'I know it is possible to be strong.'

Stress

'I know how to relax.'

'I like to exercise to relieve stress.'

'I can change situations that cause stress.'

'I am important.'

'I release stress.'

'I eat regular meals.'

'I identify stress and release it.'

'I like people.'

'People like me.'

'Success is mine.'

Studying

'I want success.'

'I know how to schedule time to study.'

'I like to study.'

'I know how to relax in tests.'

'My mind absorbs information with ease.'

'I remember what I study.'

'I remember the right answers in tests.'

Success

'I understand the Creator's definition of success.'

'I understand what it feels like to be successful.'

'I know what success is.'

'I know how to be successful in the highest and best way.'

'I know the Creator's perspective on success.'

'I know it is possible to be successful.'

Support

'I understand the Creator's definition of having support.'

'I understand what it feels like to have support.'

'I know what support is.'

'I know how to be supported in the highest and best way.'

'I know how to live my daily life with support.'

'I know the Creator's perspective on support.'

'I know it is possible to be supported.'

Teaching

'I understand the Creator's definition of teaching others.'

'I understand what it feels like to teach others.'

'I know how to teach others in the highest and best way.'

'I know the Creator's perspective on teaching.'

'I know it is possible to teach others.'

Time Management

'I know how to plan my time wisely.'

'I know how to create quiet time without interruptions.'

'I have plenty of time.'

'I am the master of my schedule.'

'I know how to start with today and plan for tomorrow.'

'Planning gives me more fun time.'

'I am flexible and persistent.'

'I recognize and deal with conflicting time demands.'

'It is always possible.'

'I know how to set my own priorities.'

'Planning gives me maximum benefits from minimum time.'

'I take action steps now.'

'I am confident in my judgement and priorities.'

Understanding

'I understand the Creator's definition of understanding.'

'I understand what it feels like to understand others.'

'I know what understanding is.'

'I know how to understand others in the highest and best way.'

'I know how to live my daily life understanding.'

'I know the Creator's perspective on understanding.'

'I know it is possible to understand.'

Unity

'I understand the Creator's definition of unity.'

'I understand what unity feels like.'

'I know what unity is.'

'I know the Creator's perspective on unity.'

Upliftment

'I understand the Creator's definition of being uplifted.'

'I understand what it feels like to uplift myself and others.'

'I know how to uplift myself and others.'

'I know how to live my daily life uplifting myself and others in the highest and best way.'

'I know the Creator's perspective on uplifting myself and others.'

'I know it is possible to uplift myself and others.'

Value

'I understand the Creator's definition of the value of all things.'

'I understand what it feels like to have value.'

'I know what value is.'

'I know how to live my daily life valuing life.'

'I know the Creator's perspective on value.'

'I know it is possible to have value.'

Versatility

'I understand the Creator's definition of versatility.'

'I understand what it feels like to be versatile.'

'I know what versatility is.'

'I know how to be versatile in the highest and best way.'

'I know the Creator's perspective on versatility.'

'I know it is possible to be versatile.'

Vision

'I understand the Creator's definition of being a visionary.'

'I understand what it feels like to have vision.'

'I know how to be a visionary in the highest and best way.'

'I know how to live my daily life full of foresight.'

'I know the Creator's perspective on being a visionary.'

'I know it is possible to be a visionary.'

Weight Loss

'I take responsibility for what I eat.'

'I see myself as attractive and thin.'

'I enjoy fruit and vegetables.'

'I enjoy exercise.'

'I know how to exercise.'

'I enjoy eating less.'

'I understand what it feels like to eat less.'

'I know how to eat less.'

'I know how to live my daily life eating less.'

'I know it is possible to eat less.'

'I understand the definition of eating healthily.'

'I understand what it feels like to eat healthily.'

'I know how to eat healthily.'

'I know how to live my daily life eating healthily.'

'I know the Creator's perspective on eating healthily.'

'I know it is possible to eat healthily.'

'I understand the Creator's definition of being attractive and thin.'

'I understand what it feels like to be attractive and thin.'

'I know it is possible to be attractive and thin.'

'I understand the Creator's definition of weight loss.'

'I understand what it feels like to lose weight.'

'I know how to lose weight.'

'I understand what it feels like to lose weight daily.'

'I understand what it feels like to exercise.'

'I know how to exercise responsibly.'

'I know how to live my daily life exercising.'

'I know it is possible to exercise.'

'I understand what it feels like to replace eating with exercise.'

'I understand how to feel good about myself.'

'I understand what it feels like to eat food that is good for my body.'

'I know how to live my daily life without overeating.'

'I know how to live my daily life without being discouraged about my weight.'

Worry

'It does no good to worry.'

'Worries vanish from my mind.'

'I understand what it feels like to be free from worry.'

'I know how to live my daily life without worry.'

'I know it is possible to live without worry.'

'I understand what it feels like to have a healthy outlook on life.'

'I understand what it feels like not to permit others to bring me down.'

'I understand what it feels like never to give up.'

'I understand how to live my life full of goodness and hope.'

'I understand what it feels like to be a responsible person.'

'I understand what it feels like to believe in myself.'

'I understand what it feels like to be respected by others.'

'I understand what it feels like to have fortitude and wisdom.'

'I understand what it feels like to receive productive and positive thoughts from the Creator daily.'

'I know it is possible for my known and unknown senses to seek positive feelings.'

'I understand how to have balance in all aspects of my life.'

'I understand the difference between concern and worry.'

'I understand what it feels like to view the future in a positive light.'

'I understand what it feels like to be infused with positive thinking.'

'I understand what it feels like to be at one with life past, present and future.'

'I understand what it feels like to control my destiny through the Creator of All That Is.'

26

DNA 3 PRE-REQUISITES

These are the pre-requisites for utilizing the DNA 3 information. These guidelines and exercises should be followed and practised every day.

Remember the Healer is the Creator of All That Is

Always remember that the true healer is the Creator of All That Is. Our job as healers is to listen and love the people we are working with, to pray for them and witness the Creator of All That Is doing the healing. If you are motivated by anything other than a reverence for all of creation and a profound love of the Creator of All That Is, you will limit yourself.

Accept the Healing

The acceptance of a healing by both the practitioner and the client is necessary for the healing to take place.

Love the People

Your prime directive as a healer is to love all the people who come to you, while maintaining proper discernment of the truth and of yourself.

Witness the Healing

The practitioner's job is to be a witness to the healing from the Creator of All That Is and to know how to recognize when this healing has occurred. Witnessing a physical healing, reprogramming a belief or teaching a feeling are all healings. Reprogramming a person's belief system so that they know they are worthy of the Creator's love is a healing in itself. Teaching a person how to love themselves is also a healing. The validity of reprogramming is evident from the differences witnessed in people's daily lives.

Make a Commitment

Make a commitment to follow through with this work. Make a commitment to master the planes of existence. Be committed to practising ThetaHealing. Be committed to doing your best. Allow yourself to know that you've earned the right to do this work.

Live in Joy

Radiate the energy of joy outward to the world! Feel the giggles of joy throughout your body! Know the Creator of All That Is protects you and you are now impervious to evil; it cannot attach itself to you. You are free to radiate the power of God's joy and love.

Practise Remote Viewing

Practise going inside the body and exploring the different systems until you are comfortable with it and accurate at it. Practise remote viewing long distance.

Do Readings Every Day

Practice is key.

Do Readings Without Anger

Compulsive anger will block you from getting the desired result in a reading. If you are angry, then something inside you is not getting what you want or need. As the healer, you are required to find out why you are angry with yourself or someone else. Step out of the room and quickly do belief or feeling work on yourself. Your anger with another person may be a reflection of your anger towards yourself.

You have the challenge of staying in a good space in spite of these situations. It is important to be grounded, back in your body, cleaned up and in a good mood by the end of the day.

Remember Everyone Is in Their Own Paradigm

Practise readings and healings on others so you get used to going out of your own paradigm and going into another person's paradigm. Remember, what you *think* is reality isn't really going on at all. When you go into another person's space, you are interacting with their paradigm, *their* world, throughout the reading, not yours. Always ask the Creator to let you see them from the highest and best perspective.

You may see that they want to keep their sickness. As the healer, your job is to not judge them, but to ask them, 'How is this serving you?'

Take Action

Without action, nothing happens. There is a distinct difference between thinking about doing something (procrastinating) and actually doing it, both physically and metaphysically.

Manipulate Time

Remember that time is under the Law of Gravity, one of the easier Laws to bend. It is an illusion. Witnessing an instant healing is an example of bending time. Practise going above your space to command time to last longer or to go faster.

By learning how to manipulate time, you are able to break from the inherited illusion that life is controlling you and you are merely a participant in whatever it has to offer. In truth, our lives are a reflection of our own paradigm, our own creation. We can actually go out of our paradigm, command what we want to create in our life and allow it to happen.

Experience the Planes

Go up to the Seventh Plane and ask to experience the different planes of existence through the Seventh Plane, with the Creator as your guide. This will keep you from being distracted by the brain candy of the planes and provide you with a clear perspective of each plane. Stay focused.

Manifest Change in your Life

What do you want to change in your life? What do you want to have happen in the next year? You can manifest optimal health or a soulmate, or ask for a financial situation to become the way you choose it to be. Remember, you create your own reality.

Persevere!!!

Just keep going…

Send a Dream

Go above your space and send someone a dream. This is best done at 3 A.M., which is when the person will be most open to it. They will dream that they are talking to you.

Holding, sending or returning from a dream will teach you how to control time in the astral plane.

Be Open to Learning New Abilities

This will help you be open to bringing change into your life.

Send a Positive Thought to a Specific Person

Go above your space and send someone a positive thought. (You will need to get validation that they have received the thought form you have sent to them.)

Programme Yourself So That Everyone You Work with Will Feel Good and Happy

If you have this programme, your clients will want to come back. Some healers don't like sick people; some don't like people in general. So test yourself for programmes of 'I hate people' or 'I hate sick people'.

With Power Comes Responsibility...

Be careful with your thoughts! Be aware of what you are doing with your manifestations! *The more you are in Theta, the more what you think will show up in your life.* So be clear about what you want, don't sell yourself short and always ask for the highest and best. If you want money, for example, ask to receive it in the highest and best way. If you want success, be clear about what kind of success you want. If you ask for patience, the Creator of All That Is will give you people who will require patience. If you ask to see truth, perhaps the truth may not be what you want to see. If you ask for an instant healing, then the Creator of All That Is will keep you in the situation until it happens, so ask for it the highest and best way.

Don't Get Attached

Expect a healing, but do not be attached to the outcome. It is the Creator who is the healer, so give up the outcome. Say to your client, 'I witnessed the Creator of All That Is working with you. Let's see what happens.' If you don't achieve the results you want, it indicates that there is more belief work to be done.

Live in the Now

Many people live their lives in the past, in the future or in a delusion. A person may not be conscious that they're having a wonderful time with you until they remember it the next day!

As spiritual beings, we often find the reality of this world difficult. We attempt to escape it and in so doing miss being in the here and now. But all healing starts in the present, even if we go into other realms during the course of the healing.

Be Thankful That You Are Alive

Reaffirm that you are thankful every day. Breathe the air, watch the clouds and appreciate the life that is all around you.

Believe, Know, Live

First *believe* that a healing can happen, then *know* it can happen and then *live* its essence.

Work on Yourself!

The more belief work you do on yourself, the faster your healing abilities will improve and the fewer blocks you'll have in the process of becoming an effective healer.

Learn and grow from interaction with others and be gentle and encouraging with yourself, because you're going where you've never gone before…

Allow Yourself to Live in 'Seventh-Plane Knowingness'

Learn how to live without fear and anger and in Seventh-Plane knowingness, knowing that everything is going to be OK and that the Creator is available to you.

Our goal is to achieve Seventh-Plane consciousness.

27

VIANNA'S SAYINGS

'Talk to the Creator every day.'

'Thank the Creator every day.'

'Honour life in all its forms.'

'All is not what it seems.'

'Thoughts move faster than light. They have essence, so be careful what you think.'

'Do something to be proud of every day.'

'Slow down and notice the air and the light. Appreciate life.'

'Action is all-important.'

'It's a piece of cake.'

'It just is.'

'Whenever possible, hurt no one and nothing.'

'See the truth in people and still love them.'

'Healers go through a process: first we believe, then we know, then we live.'

'So much of our time is wasted upon useless thought forms. We must learn to focus and direct our thought-energy to the divine consciousness.'

'Live your life as if there were no secrets. Live life as an open book, so that you could tell anyone what you did today.'

'Sometimes the best secrets are kept by sharing them with the world.'

'You can love all people – including the mean ones – as long as you are connected to the Creator.'

'Prophetic power is using the power of the universe.'

'Reality is always there waiting for us to acknowledge it. It is only when you believe in reality that it becomes real on a personal level.'

'Most of the problems that occur in this existence are caused by the illusion that we are separate from the Creator.'

Afterword

by Guy Stibal

In the present day, there are literally millions of people searching for spiritual answers through information that for perhaps the first time in history is accessible to humanity to such an extent as to be overwhelming. The everyday person now has access to alternative literature on a scale that would have been unthinkable 100 or even 50 years ago. Ancient belief systems, those that are resurfacing from the collective consciousness and those that are divine, are all at our fingertips.

As searchers for spiritual knowledge, we do not realize the incredible freedom that we now have. It is our responsibility to treasure this freedom and make good use of information that for centuries was jealously guarded by individuals, passed on via word of mouth and only rarely written down, to be promptly hidden by secret societies from those who might misuse it.

Because of this influx of knowledge from many different traditions and modalities, a great smorgasbord is laid out before us, and we must be careful not to get spiritual indigestion. It might be best to learn and digest a belief system thoroughly before moving on to the next exploration. With any type of spiritual knowledge, a good dose of common sense is as sweet as any honey. We should never forget that the freedoms that we now enjoy could perhaps lead to over-stimulation, and perhaps egotism.

Altruism and good judgement should light our way forward in all matters, and this includes energy healing. If we want to be respected for our practices, then our practices must be respectable. *In order for any belief system to stand the test of time, it must be permitted to form in purity, and it must remain pure and unchanged long enough to make a shift in the consciousness of humankind.* If these spiritual teachings are to remain divine, it is necessary that they transcend the view of the mind that *rational intellect* is the supreme authority of reality. The purity of these kinds of rare mystical knowledge can then become a gnosis within – an ignition of enlightenment that emphasizes and accentuates the numinous experience with a clarity and directness that resonates with us to the very core of our being. We can then feel a deep resonance with these kinds of knowledge that at some point easily transcends the dictates of reason and is accepted by the conscious mind as truth without conflict.

ABOUT THE AUTHOR

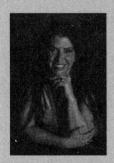 **Vianna Stibal** is a young grandmother, an artist and a writer. Her natural charisma and compassion for those in need of help have also led to her being known as a healer, intuitive and teacher.

After being taught how to connect with the Creator to co-create and facilitate the unique process called ThetaHealing, Vianna knew that she must share this gift with as many people as she could. It was this love and appreciation for the Creator and humanity that allowed her to develop the ability to see clearly into the human body and witness many instant healings.

Her encyclopaedic knowledge of the body's systems and deep understanding of the human psyche, based on her own experience as well as the insight given to her by the Creator, makes Vianna the perfect practitioner of this amazing technique. She has successfully worked with such medical challenges as hepatitis C, Epstein-Barr virus, AIDS, herpes, various types of cancers and many other disorders, diseases and genetic defects.

Vianna knows that the ThetaHealing technique is teachable, but beyond that she knows that it *needs* to be taught. She conducts seminars all over the world to teach people of all races, beliefs and religions. She has trained teachers and practitioners who are working in 14 countries, but her work will not stop there! She is committed to spreading this healing paradigm throughout the world.

www.thetahealing.com

Further Information

THETAHEALING CLASSES

ThetaHealing® is an energy-healing modality founded by Vianna Stibal, based in Ammon, Idaho, with certified instructors around the world. The classes and books of ThetaHealing are designed as therapeutic guides to developing the ability of the mind to heal.

Classes taught by Vianna and certified ThetaHealing instructors:
(A manual is given in every class)

> Basic ThetaHealing® Course
>
> Advanced ThetaHealing® Course
>
> ThetaHealing® Intuitive Anatomy Course
>
> ThetaHealing® Rainbow Children's Course
>
> ThetaHealing® Manifesting and Abundance Course
>
> ThetaHealing® Diseases and Disorders Course
>
> ThetaHealing® World Relations Course
>
> ThetaHealing® DNA 3

Certification classes taught exclusively by Vianna at the ThetaHealing Institute of Knowledge®:
(A manual is given in every class)

> Basic ThetaHealing® Instructor's Course
>
> Advanced ThetaHealing® Instructor's Course
>
> ThetaHealing® Intuitive Anatomy Instructor's Course
>
> ThetaHealing® Rainbow Children's Instructor's Course
>
> ThetaHealing® Diseases and Disorders Instructor's Course
>
> ThetaHealing® World Relations Instructor's Course
>
> ThetaHealing® DNA 3 Instructor's Course

BOOKS

Titles currently available:

ThetaHealing® (Hay House, 2010)

ThetaHealing®: *Diseases and Disorders* (Hay House, 2011)

❖❖❖❖❖

For further information about schedules for ThetaHealing® classes, please contact:

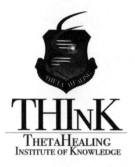

THInK
THETAHEALING
INSTITUTE OF KNOWLEDGE

All ThetaHealing and Teaching activities are now carried out at and under the auspices of the Institute, which is located at 1615 Curlew Drive, Ammon, Idaho 83406.
Tel. (office): (1) (208) 524-0808
Fax: (1) (208) 524-3061
E-mail: vianna@thetahealing.com
Website: **www.thetahealing.com**

We hope you enjoyed this Hay House book. If you'd like to
receive our online catalog featuring additional information
on Hay House books and products, or if you'd like to find out
more about the Hay Foundation, please contact:

Hay House, Inc., P.O. Box 5100, Carlsbad, CA 92018-5100
(760) 431-7695 or (800) 654-5126
(760) 431-6948 (fax) or (800) 650-5115 (fax)
www.hayhouse.com® • **www.hayfoundation.org**

❖❖❖❖❖

Published and distributed in Australia by: Hay House Australia Pty. Ltd.,
18/36 Ralph St., Alexandria NSW 2015
Phone: 612-9669-4299 • *Fax:* 612-9669-4144 • www.hayhouse.com.au

Published and distributed in the United Kingdom by: Hay House UK, Ltd.,
Astley House, 33 Notting Hill Gate, London W11 3JQ
Phone: 44-20-3675-2450 • *Fax:* 44-20-3675-2451 • www.hayhouse.co.uk

Published and distributed in the Republic of South Africa by:
Hay House SA (Pty), Ltd., P.O. Box 990, Witkoppen 2068
Phone/Fax: 27-11-467-8904 • www.hayhouse.co.za

Published in India by: Hay House Publishers India, Muskaan Complex,
Plot No. 3, B-2, Vasant Kunj, New Delhi 110 070
Phone: 91-11-4176-1620 • *Fax:* 91-11-4176-1630 • www.hayhouse.co.in

Distributed in Canada by: Raincoast, 9050 Shaughnessy St.,
Vancouver, B.C. V6P 6E5 • *Phone:* (604) 323-7100
Fax: (604) 323-2600 • www.raincoast.com

❖❖❖❖❖

Take Your Soul on a Vacation

Visit **www.HealYourLife.com**® to regroup, recharge, and reconnect
with your own magnificence.Featuring blogs, mind-body-spirit news,
and life-changing wisdom from Louise Hay and friends.

Visit **www.HealYourLife.com** today!

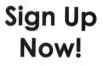